Cont

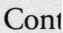

Part 1	1
Chapter 1	3
Part 2	27
Chapter 2	29
Chapter 3	37
Chapter 4	42
Chapter 5	48
Chapter 6	52
Chapter 7	62
Chapter 8	66
Chapter 9	71
Chapter 10	80
Chapter 11	84
Part 3	87
Chapter 12	89
Chapter 13	103
Chapter 14	112
Chapter 15	115
Chapter 16	121
Chapter 17	135
Chapter 18	140
Chapter 19	146
Chapter 20	158
Chapter 21	167

Chapter 22	180
Chapter 23	193
Chapter 24	202
Chapter 25	212
Chapter 26	222
Chapter 27	227
Chapter 28	233
Chapter 29	241
Chapter 30	246
Chapter 31	251
Chapter 32	257
Chapter 33	260
Afterword	269
Acknowledgements	281
Photo credits	282

Part 1

Part 1

1

Groundhog Day, number 19. I pulled back the curtains and there was the bright blue sky, a few puffballs of white cloud, the ever-green treetops completely still. *Simpsons* weather, the aviators call it, and that's what you get day after day out there. The rain will sweep through in the afternoon, water the plants, clear the air, then head on inland and hand back the blue sky. But this is how it starts every morning. Leighton Buzzard, it is not.

It's why I had chosen to get my pilot's licence in Florida. Back home, you could spend a whole month in flight school waiting for the rain to lift. And I only had a month to play with, kill some time usefully. Then the serious business was to begin. At last, a chance to do my bit for Queen and Country. Seven years with the military, all that technical training, all that lung-bursting effort, and I had made it into one of the best military units in the world. Now, it was time for the real thing and I was gunning to repay some of the investment in me. I hadn't stopped thinking about it from the moment the rumour of deployment raced around the regiment. There'd been a little extra adrenaline in the blood every day, all day.

I looked again at Trig's text from last night. *It's on. Official. We're deploying. Get yourself back to UK soon.*

Now that I knew I wouldn't be waking him in the middle of the night, I replied: *They told me. Brilliant. Finally. All good here. Just a few more hours' solo to go. See you in a couple of days.*

Then back into the clockwork daily routine – out of the shower, a shave and into the khaki cargo shorts, side pockets for wallet and phone, a fresh black cotton T-shirt, suede hiking trainers, wraparound military-style anti-glare shades, beige baseball cap, basic rubber digital watch. It would be the same tomorrow, and the day after – and then something a bit warmer for the flight home and the grey skies of Leighton Buzzard. I laid out the running kit at the foot of the bed – for later, once I was done flying and the air had cooled.

I like routine, order, method, punctuality, clarity. It's one of the reasons I had taken to military life so eagerly. I don't like mess, chaos, bad timekeeping, confusion, vagueness. I'm not OCD, just tidy. Maybe it's to do with the drive to sort myself out after the shambles of my teenage years. I am restless. I like a change of scene. I need it. But in between the changes, when I'm in the new place, I like Groundhog Day, to know where I'm at, know what each day's going to bring.

I sent Mum a text, apologising for not calling last night but would do so before my ten-miler and before she had settled down for *Songs of Praise*.

Down in the communal kitchen, it was Scene 2 from Groundhog Day: bowl of porridge and honey, banana, mug of tea, milky, no sugar. A few of the other flight-school students were milling about and we exchanged the usual pleasantries and mild banter. I was going to miss these guys, this downtime. Compared to SAS training, 'P' Company with the Paras and the Cambrian Patrols, learning to fly was a breeze, especially in the Sunshine State. We'd had a great few weeks and, united in the same experience, we had formed a bit of a bond.

During the day we had the buzz of flying and some hard study, and in the evenings it was barbecues, cards, movies, occasionally a trip to the beach or out to a bar and, best of all so far, to Cape Canaveral to see the Shuttle launch. We'd had fun, and that was exactly what I needed after a couple of years living in swamps, jungles, desert and frozen mountains, lying filthy in foxholes and shitting into plastic bags. And it was exactly what I needed before deploying to the deadliest theatre of war on the planet.

This part of Florida is like an advert for the American Dream – quiet closes with large, timber-clad family homes, manicured gardens, SUVs in the drive, basketball hoops over the garage. I slid on my shades, tugged down my baseball cap and pulled the door to. It was already simmering hot, just like it was every morning at that time, and moms and dads were piling their children into cars for a day out, probably to the beach. There's a lot of beach here, on and on in both directions as far as I could see from a thousand feet up. I exchanged the customary Good Mornings and nods. Groundhog Day. I probably had two, maybe three more Groundhog Days to go. I was going to miss the pleasant routine of it all.

Through the thick band of pines and evergreen oaks, I could hear the thwack of clubs on golf balls followed by – Groundhog Day – the whoops of approval and groans of despair. It was only a ten-minute stroll alongside the golf course, but I was sweating hard by the time I ducked into the short path through the woods past the clubhouse. Rico the barman was out the back having his crafty smoke.

'Hey man, how you doing? You dropping in for your club sandwich later?'

'Why not? I might just do that – for a change. See how I am set after flying.'

'You must be almost done with your lessons, yeah?'

'Yep, almost there now. I'm going to miss your place.'

'We're going to miss you too, man. Take it easy, English guy.'

'Yeah, you too.'

I walked through the club car park, straight into Hangar Way and past the peeling driftwood sign, all the aircraft lined up on the big apron outside their hangars, neat as houses, one taxiing in, one taxiing out. Overhead, a few in the pattern, circling and circling, getting their hours in.

The star-shaped runways wobbled in the rising heat and in the far distance, to the north, sat the squat little control tower on its own, with couple of easy-going guys in there on their coffees going 'Yeah sure, November Foxtrot One Four Two Delta Tango, clear to land.' It wasn't the biggest airfield in the world. It wasn't the biggest airfield in the county. But it was laidback and friendly, and nice and cheap.

Into the nondescript flight school building, the chill of the air conditioning washing over me. The chief instructor was behind the reception desk, the VHF radio bubbling away with updates.

'Good morning, Jamie, how are you today?'

'Yeah, I'm good thanks. You?'

There were a lot of students around for that time of the morning and I asked when I might get out. Bit of a backlog but, he rubbed his chin and reckoned, they could get me up with an instructor for a check flight around ten. Then I'd just have to re-join the list and wait out for a solo flight in the afternoon.

I checked the manifest and meteorology reports – sunshine, blast of heavy rain, more sunshine – and headed upstairs. I grabbed a coffee and settled at a computer. There was nothing to study any longer – I had passed all eight written exams – so I sent a couple of emails and trawled the news sites: Hurricane Dean gathering strength in the Caribbean, but it's heading towards Mexico not up the Panhandle ... Aid struggling to reach victims of a huge earthquake in Peru ... Another suicide attack in Afghanistan ... Groundhog Day there too.

One of the instructors – aviators, black jeans, short-sleeved white shirt – strolled towards me and tossed me the keys. It was around ten.

'Hey, buddy, you're on. We're in November Foxtrot Five Five Two Yankee Tango.'

We strode out to our plane, not saying much, just pulling on our bottles of water. I had gone solo about a week earlier and this was a check flight to make sure I hadn't got complacent or picked up bad habits. It must be boring for the instructor once a student is up and running, just working through his hours. There's no fun kicking tyres, watching a guy check the fuel's not been contaminated. Then once you're in the air, staring out the window at the same view, hour after hour, day after day. Me, I just wanted to get some more time down in the logbook. But we were fine and friendly enough.

The plane was tiny, just 20-foot long, and from the flight school it looked like a toy plane you'd find on a fairground ride. I was almost taller than it. 'Gorgeous little aircraft,' said the instructor as he patted it. 'Thinking of getting one. Cute little commuter. Beats the shit out of sitting on the highway.'

My adrenaline was starting to flow because I was about to get airborne and I was *that* close to being a qualified pilot. We did the pre-flight check walkaround, him looking at me looking at the aircraft. I pulled the aileron flaps up and down, waggled the rudder, ran my hand over the propeller shafts, peered down at the tyres and the suspension system, nodded my head a lot with a serious face. Frankly, unless the tail rudder's hanging off or the prop has got a load of rope tangled in it, you're not going to have a clue if the aircraft is airworthy. The real business is to be found in the engine and that's for the ground-crew engineers. The walkaround is an essential procedure, but doing it as an unqualified rookie, even after as many hours as I'd done, you're hoping the instructor is looking as hard as you are, just in case. You're just feeling cool in your shades, pumped about hitting the skies.

It was getting seriously hot and the asphalt was giving off some extra heat. The sweat was running from scalp to toe. We went to check the fuel, make sure no impurities had found their way into the tank. I took out the tiny transparent cup from my flight kitbag, got down under the belly of the fuselage, opened up the fuel-tank cap and held the cup under the little T-valve, a little like you find on a winebox. Out came a dash of low-lead blue and I came out from underneath and held it up to the light. It was mild blue and clear, no contaminants.

Regulations say you're meant to transfer it into another receptacle and dispose of it safely, but all the instructors flicked their head to say *Just toss it*. It was barely an eggcup's worth and the moment it hit the asphalt, it shimmered and bubbled and then it was gone. Fair play because that amount of fuel isn't going to burn down a blue tit's bedside table. The full 110 litres in the tank is another matter. I pulled out the oil dipstick behind the flap over the engine. All fine.

'Okay, Jamie, up we go.'

I pulled out the wooden chocks from the wheels and laid them to one side. He handed me the key and I went around the prop towards the left of the aircraft and the captain's seat; he climbed into the right-hand seat. I squeezed in and ran through all the pre-flight instrument checks, got cleared by the tower and rolled out to the holding area, and then – loved that feeling – the wheels were away from the asphalt and we were climbing, Florida coast stretching further and further.

We ran a few patterns around the airfield, practised a couple of touch-and-goes and finished off with a run up to Flagler County airport about 15 miles to the north. It was pretty quiet in the cockpit. There was not much to say. I had a lot of hours in the bank, dual and solo. When you start it's not non-stop chatter on the two-way. But my confidence was good now. It was just a question of perfecting the routines and techniques. Flying is all about planning, careful checking and procedure, not a great deal different to the challenges of learning to drive a car. It's not a gift some are born with, some not. Everyone just has to learn the procedures, then keep practising.

Landing was my favourite element of the flight because it was the most challenging. First, you have to get the approach right, then use the flaps to scrub off airspeed and keep her level. You've got to be right on the money and get the balance just right: too fast and it's hard to control, too slow and you risk stalling. I was cruising at about 70 knots downwind when I got on the comms and thumbed the pressel switch on the control stick between my legs.

'Ormond Tower, Ormond Tower, this is November Five Five Two Yankee Tango.'

The laid-back southern drawl crackled through my headset: 'November Five Five Two Yankee Tango, go ahead.'

I asked permission for a full-stop landing and was given the all-clear. Turning into the wind, I reduced power a little and began dropping altitude. There was a little more bump on the wings as I pulled back on the throttle and the aircraft pitched forward. It's only a gentle dip but it feels as if the nose has dropped sharply. You have been looking at the artificial horizon indicator on the instrument panel then suddenly it's the real horizon looming up at you and it's a weird sensation. I kept easing off the throttle and adjusting the trim, holding her steady at about 55 knots. Less than 50 and you're going to drop out.

Before the threshold point – the beginning of the runway – I lined up the nose with the dotted lines, gently scrubbing off more speed by lowering the flaps. It was getting bumpier and bumpier just as it does on a commercial aircraft when you land. At about

25 feet, I powered off and pulled back the stick and the aircraft flared.

'Stall! Stall!' The strong southern accent of the electronic warning screamed through the headset. But I had got used to the shock of that by then. You don't want to hear that when you're 1,000 feet up but when you are about to touch down, it's good. It means you have cut the power in time and you are gliding in now.

The rear wheels thumped on to the asphalt as one, and I pulled the stick back into my belly to flare, feet straight on the pedals. I lurched forward as the nose wheel dropped down, held back the stick a little and started feathering the brakes with tugs on the finger switch. I slowed to a jogging pace and rolled her back to the apron. The instructor turned, gave me a thumbs-up sign and yawned. Another hour in the logbook.

Back in the building, the flight manager said he'd probably be able to get me up for another run around lunchtime. I grabbed a bottle of water, chatted to a few other students and went back to one of the computer terminals. With no theory exams to study for, the hanging around between flights was getting tedious. The flight-school office building was pretty basic and functional, no frills or diversions, and it was way too hot to go for a walk. There was virtually nothing to do but drum fingers and wait.

It was close to lunch, about one o'clock, when I got the nod. The club sandwich would have to wait. I drained my second bottle of water and went to the restroom. I splashed water over my face and neck and mop of thick dark hair, stared at myself in the mirror. Ronnie, the Regimental Sergeant Major, would certainly have a few choice words for me when we mustered at the reserve London base for pre-deployment. Something along the lines of *We're not going on fooking holiday, mate!* I'd have to get all that cut off as soon I got home. But I was in top shape still, pleased I'd kept up my fitness levels, run daily, and kept the beers and burgers to a minimum. I was looking good, feeling good. I was going to hit the ground running.

. . .

Okay, from here I'm going to tell it to you in real time, the present, because whenever I think about it – and I do many times every day – it feels like it's happening again. When I'm telling someone about it, it's like I am right there, not just thinking about it … it feels like I'm living it all over again, that it's happening right now. My skin actually prickles. The intensity of it. It's as big an experience as a man can have, and live to tell the tale. It only took 45 seconds. You can take all the other experiences in my life before and after and compress them down tight as you like, but these 45 seconds are still bigger than all of them put together …

So, I head out of the cool of the flight school into the furnace of the midday heat, the whole airfield wobbling in a thick haze. I zero towards the plane, the only one out there, callsign November Five Five Zero X-ray Lima – written as N550XL – emblazoned in blue on the white fuselage. You rarely go up in the same aircraft twice in a day. That isn't a particularly big deal but each aircraft, like each instructor, does have its own character and slight idiosyncrasies.

There are about 20 aircraft in all at the flight school, three of them the model I've been training in from the off. It's the only aircraft I have flown. It seems to be doing the job for me but I couldn't tell you if it is an easy or difficult plane to fly.

I do the walkaround, check the fuel and oil, move aside the chocks. Using the handle on the fuselage I yank myself on to the wing, unlock the door and lower myself into the seat. It's hot as a greenhouse in there and I can smell the last student pilot. There's about the same room in the fibreglass cockpit as you have in a regular saloon car. The seat's a bit wider maybe but my head is no more than three inches from the roof. I adjust the seat so that my feet are comfortable on the rudder pedals. I take out the headset from my flight kit on the passenger seat, plug it and turn on the ATIS – the automatic terminal information service. I dial to the correct frequency. The broadcast is on a loop, giving updates on the weather, runway availability and so on. I'll keep this on the whole time because, if a potential hazard materialises, like a sudden change in the weather or a problem at an airfield, a notice goes out to all pilots in the airspace. I set my altimeter.

The basics of flying are contained in the mnemonic FREDA – fuel, radio, engine, direction and altitude – and this procedure is drilled into you from the start. You run through those checks over and over when you are in the air and there is strict procedure on the ground too. I flick on the mains switch and the instrument panel bursts into life, display lights on, needles quivering. I turn the Alpha and Bravo magnetos on and off to check the electrical current is good. I run through all instrument panel checks and get on the radio.

'Ormond Tower, Ormond Tower, this is November Five Five Zero X-ray Lima.'

'November Five Five Zero X-ray Lima, go ahead.'

I tell them I'm on the apron and ask permission to taxi out to the holding areas for the active runway, the one pointing into the prevailing wind. No problem, I'm clear to move out.

The vertical glass door above my head is still open and I shout 'clear prop' even though there is no one within 200 yards. It sounds dumb, but the tight discipline of procedure is vital. Accidents happen when people get lazy or complacent and start cutting corners. I pull down the door and secure my airman's pocket wallet around my knees with the Velcro straps, the map of my airspace clearly visible through the clear plastic cover.

I take a 360-degree look around the aircraft and turn the key in the ignition, just like you do in a car. The engine splutters into life and a light shudder runs through the fuselage. The throttle is in the centre column on my right and I give it the gentlest push. I can feel the aircraft pulling a little, but I hold her firm with the two little finger brakes on the throttle stick.

I take one more look around and release the brakes. The aircraft is barely moving so I give it a little boost and get her up to jogging pace, steering with the rudder pedals. I am looking around, checking for hazards, left and right at junctions, just as you do out on the roads. It's very quiet and I bump along the main taxiway to the first holding area, apply the brakes, and run through my final checks.

I power up to about 4,000rpm, not full whack but enough to know the engine will get me in the air with no obvious signs of distress. I am squeezing the brakes manually on the finger switches and the aircraft starts straining hard, desperate to get going. It's an exciting moment. Experienced pilots tell me they still get the same rush after 20 years. All that power and energy tensing aircraft and pilot, the knowledge that in a minute or so you'll be defying gravity, up there with the birds high above the earth. That if you screw it up, or it screws you up, well …

I throttle off and taxi out to the final holding area next to the start of active runway 35 – short for the 350 degrees of the circle at which it points. I relay my position to the tower and tell them I am ready to get airborne. If an aircraft is coming in to land, they ask you to hold, but not today. A lazy voice clears me for take-off.

There's no hanging about now. I roll her forward and turn the nose into the wind, the front wheel lined up straight down the middle of the long runway. I knock off the brakes and start pushing the throttle forward. I am aiming to hit 55 knots (63mph) and I am watching the needle of the airspeed indicator nudge around the dial. I push the throttle right the way forward, my left hand taking up the slack on the control stick until I feel it bite but not take, balancing the rudder pedals to keep her dead centre.

I hit 55 knots after about 250 yards and I start pulling back the control stick. You have to trust the science. At 55, in an aircraft of this weight, you have the optimum amount of speed and lift to get off the ground. The wheels peel away from the asphalt and there is only air beneath us. It is the critical point and I pull the stick back a little further – not too much or I'll scrub airspeed, climb too steeply and risk stalling. It's all a balance, like patting your head, rubbing your stomach and tapping your feet all at once. The thrill and the fear are felt in the stomach and the back of the mouth.

Straightaway, new dynamic forces, different laws of physics get to work on the aircraft. There is pressure on the wings and the torque pulls the aircraft left because the prop is spinning clockwise, the other way. It is Newton's third law: 'for every action, there is an equal and opposite reaction'. To counter it, I press down the right rudder pedal and the plane straightens up. I am at full power, the throttle right forward, but I'm resisting the instinct to pull back too hard on the stick. I want to keep that steady angle but put some distance over the bank of woods at the end of the runway. Not too steep, not too shallow, full power but not too much stick.

The climb seems greater from inside the cockpit than when viewed from the ground. The dead flat landscape opens up rapidly to my left, the Atlantic Ocean to my right, straight ahead of me only the instrument panel. Learning to fly, it takes time to get accustomed to not looking out of a windscreen. You're travelling blind, wholly reliant on the efficiency of the dials and displays.

I am climbing, climbing, heading for 1,000 feet when I can get into the pattern, the engine driving the prop, the prop pulling in the air and spewing it out behind, just as a boat propeller does with water. The altimeter tells me I have reached my ceiling and I pull back on the power, push the stick forward and level out, trimming the pitch. I call up the tower and give them my position and tell them I plan to run a few circuits. Then maybe I'll head up to Flagler and execute a touch-and-go. I'll see.

I'm on an air road, heading down a long straight, then I bank left and, below me, there are the never-ending beach, the golf courses, the lovely manicured housing estates among the woods, sun bouncing off the Halifax and Tomoka rivers and a thousand creeks like veins in the earth's skin, the aircraft at the flight school like toys on a kid's playmat. The air's a bit cooler up here and cruising at 70 knots there's a bit of a through draught. It is a beautiful sight and a beautiful feeling.

I do a few laps and execute a couple of touch-and-go landings. When I request permission to make a full-stop landing, the tower tells me the runway is busy so I stay up in the pattern. My stomach is rumbling a little and I am looking forward to my sandwich over at the clubhouse, nestled down there in the cool of the woods. I come around the circuit and I'm downwind. I give the controllers my position and they tell me I'm clear to come in. I look out of the side window and see the pleasure boats and yachts making their way up and down the Halifax River. In the distance, the Atlantic is like a giant sheet of silver under the strong sun.

I am no happier than the day before or the day before that, but I am as happy as I have ever been in my life. I am on top of the world in every sense. It has been a long journey from my delinquent teenage years, that's for sure. When I was 16, drugs and crime were likely going to be my career, probably some jail time too. At 32, on another sunny day in Florida, USA, I feel like Superman. Maybe that's why I want to fly so badly.

From classroom layabout, street-corner scally and petty criminal, I am now an elite soldier, a mountain leader, an instructor in scuba diving, Nordic and Alpine skiing, a fully qualified paramedic, the holder of a master's degree and the speaker of four languages. I am about to add a pilot's licence to that list. At over 30, I am one of the older recruits to 21 SAS, so in a few years when my time in the military is up, who knows, I am thinking I might even become a commercial pilot. Or maybe open my own diving school or launch my own expedition business. I used to have no prospects, now I have too many options.

I am very proud of turning around my life, but I'm not one to boast. I am not like that. I just want to explain quite how far I have come by lunchtime on 19 August 2007.

When I see the flame.

When the 45 seconds begin.

I am banking into the crosswind, looking out of the left-side canopy window, when I see it. Or I think I do. I turn my head back to the instrument panel, maybe in denial. Then straightaway I look again. Yes, that's a flame. It's yellowy-orange and it's streaking in a very thin line out of the NACA duct – the air inlet – on the front fuselage over the engine. A heavyweight has caught me unawares and punched me in the chest.

You're meant to say 'Ormond Tower, Ormond Tower, this is November Foxtrot Five Five Zero X-ray Lima' and give your position and wait for them to respond. But I just squeeze the comms and shout, 'May day! May day! Engine fire!'

I look out the window and the flame is getting longer and thicker. The tower is in my ear, all laidback and asking for details. No idea what they're saying. I have one thought: *Get this burning bastard down on the ground. Fast.*

But I can't go fast. Or I'll pile in. I have to perform a normal landing at normal speed. I'm at 1,000 feet. I figure I've got 45 seconds. I turn into wind, look out the window. Fire loves a wind. There are 12 knots of it and I'm heading into it at about 70 knots.

There's a fire extinguisher in an awkward position in the back, but so what? And no parachute in these light aircraft. Why not?

The tower is in my ear again but all I'm hearing in my head is the voice of my first instructor and his advice for an emergency. His slow southern drawl is on a loop now: 'Just fly the damn aircraft, man, just fly the damn aircraft.'

My heart is jack-hammering my chest and the torrent of adrenaline has fogged my head. Focus, focus! I want to go faster and it is an effort of will to pull back on the throttle and slow her down. The aircraft pitches forward, and there's the real horizon and there are the flames. It's not a streak any longer. It's a full fire and it's streaming down the nose, mostly down the sides rather than over, loving the wind I'm now flying straight into. Slow down, slow down! I force myself to ease off the throttle, fine-tuning the trim, keeping her at 55 knots. I am willing on the altimeter: 900 feet ... 850 feet ... 800 ...

The tower is back in my ear but the flames have penetrated the footwell, licking at the rudder pedals, and I don't give a shit what they are saying. There's a slight airflow into the cockpit through a couple of vents and the flames are greedy for it. There's no way my heart can beat harder or faster now, but I can't do anything different. It's a normal landing or a crash. Or a mid-air explosion.

Six hundred and fifty feet ... 600 ... and the flames are at my knees. I am wearing shorts but I can feel no pain. There's that much adrenaline in my blood.

My life is not flashing before me in a chronological sequence of memories. It is presented as a collage, a hundred images all at once: Mum, Dad, home, school, girlfriend Terri, Norway, scuba-diving, SAS buddies ...

Five hundred and fifty feet ... 500 ... and the flames are now above my waist. Okay, I am in a full panic now. No use pretending to myself otherwise. That is proper heat on my legs. I squeeze the pressel switch on the stick and yell: 'May day! May day!' The tower says something back. Still all laidback and drawly.

There is no smoke, that's good, but my legs are burning and the flames are stabbing at my chest. I am, quite literally, just sitting in a moving fire. I go into rapid breathing. The earth seems a long, long way away, everything still tiny.

Call it what you want: a lightbulb moment, an epiphany, divine intervention, whatever. But, in an instant, I am overwhelmed by a sense of calm. Which is weird because I'm on fire and if bookies were watching and taking odds, I'm a 5,000–1 shot on still being alive in 20 seconds. Maybe that's why I am feeling calm now. It's all over and it's going to be quick. Maybe 15 seconds of agony, then lights out. I can deal with 15 seconds of agony.

I know what I am going to do. I am going to get out and jump. Maybe just having a plan, being decisive, is feeding me the calm. Jumping without a parachute's not in the emergency protocol they teach you, but it's a better plan than sitting here on fire, rolling to a halt on the runway burned to a blackened cinder or dropping out of the sky and piling in as a fireball. I think about my calm. I am amazed by it and very impressed. How many others would be sitting there like a Buddha statue, on fire, just a few breaths of life left, calm as stone?

The control tower is at the far end of the airfield over to the left and I veer gently in that direction, about 20 degrees from the runway. I am not stupid. I am not going to jump on to asphalt. Might as well stay in the aircraft and get incinerated. The long grass will be spongy from the daily afternoon downpours. The tower asks me for an update on my situation. Like they are asking how the weather is up there. They must be watching me come in, wreathed in flame. I am heading in their direction. The flight school and hangars are ahead on my right. I squeeze the pressel switch and say, 'I don't think I'm going to make it.' I tear off the headphones and my cap and hurl them into the footwell of the passenger seat. I am aware of intense heat but I am not in pain. Weird. The human body is an amazing bit of kit.

I am now wearing the flames, and I've got ten seconds left. I am going to do this properly, as per the protocol. I turn the ignition key to off, I flick the red magneto switches Alpha and Bravo to off, the master switch to off, lights off, strobes off, fuel pump off, fuel selector valve off. I am gliding now in my own personal inferno, the prop still milling. The flames are dancing around my chin. I am calm but I am hyperventilating through the side of my mouth. I guess to keep the fire out. It isn't a decision, just a reflex.

I am controlling my direction and balance with the pedals and stick. I love this little plane. It's staying with me right to the bitter end. It's not giving up on me. Squinting through the heat – thank God for my Oakley's – I see the cross runway. I've got to clear that before I bail. Just get to the grass on the other side, then I'm out of here like Jack Rabbit. It's getting really hot, but still no pain. Maybe it's the human mind, not the body, that deserves the plaudits for this.

I am at about 50 feet doing about 40 knots when I make my move. I unbuckle the three-point harness at the waist and lean forward into the flames to wriggle my shoulders free. I go to push up the vertical canopy door, but it doesn't want to budge. The nose feels a little heavy so I pull back the stick a little. I press my palm and the underside of my arm up to the elbow against the canopy window and, pushing up with one foot, the door springs upwards. I sit back down into the flames and pull back the stick a little more, straighten her up on the rudder pedals.

I see the cross runway right in front of me and the grass beyond, but the flames are slapping my face, burning my brow and earlobes, and I have to close my eyes. I am hyperventilating furiously through a peephole at the edge of my mouth.

Now!

I clamber on to the seat and I'm over the lip of door, hands and knees, on to the left wing and into a tornado of fire, the worst pain I have ever experienced. Ever will. The backwash from the propeller has turned the fire into a giant blowtorch. I stand up at a slight angle, knees bent, and the right side of my body is melting through the muscle down to the bone. My T-shirt and shorts are incinerating, my hair is on fire, the right side of my body is blistering and bubbling like a chop under a grill on max.

I have to jump clean, like I do in para training, and land well. It can't be sloppy. The timing has to be just right. A second too early I die in the fall, a second too late I die in the blast wave and fireball. I wait a second or two and take a massive leap away from the fuselage so I'm not hit by the tail wing. I snap my knees and feet together and clap my hands into prayer position over my head.

It's a heavy fall. I have landed feet first, which is good, but the roll is sloppy, too fast. I snap over, hard down on to my right shoulder and the right of my face. Multiple areas of my body compete for the greatest amount of pain. My nose, eye socket and cheekbone have been pile-driven into my skull. My guts feel as if they have been torn open, my collarbone has popped and I am so winded I cannot get a breath in. My lungs have slapped together and are stuck.

I am on fire and I need to put out the flames. Arms flat to the side, legs together I roll from side to side and over and over. Most of the flames have gone but I'm smouldering and there is a stench of fuel and burning flesh. My right shoulder is still on fire so I slap it furiously. So is my scalp. I'm like a Roman candle and I smear my head in the grass, patting it with both hands.

Then I remember the aircraft – I have only been on the ground about four or five seconds – and I go into the foetal position, make myself as small as possible, pressing myself into the earth. I cover my face with my hands and peek through my fingers. It is about 20 metres away, nose really heavy and really, really on fire, left wing angling down, the prop about six feet from the ground. Everything now in slow motion.

Of all the intense sensory experiences convulsing me in those 45 seconds, the sound of the plane piling in – the huge crumpling – remains as vivid as any. Earth flies through the flames and the nose concertinas into the cockpit.

It's going to blow. I know that and I stare at it, utterly transfixed. It is very close to me and maybe the huge crumpling noise has made me aware of the proximity. Maybe that's why it's so vivid because now is the first time I become conscious of fear. I was too busy up in the air to be frightened. But now events are out of my control. Let's see what happens. Or not see. Not know.

I think it's about seven or eight seconds when it blows, a long time anyhow. I am the most petrified I have ever been. But I am managing to get some air in my lungs again.

Boom!

I have been in training bunkers with heavy ordnance falling above but I have never heard or felt an explosion like this. One hundred litres of low-lead blue now a massive bomb. Flames shoot up in a giant mushrooming column of flame and black smoke. The force of the shockwave, Jesus Christ. It goes straight through me like it is something solid, then comes back again. Every last ounce of air in my lungs is ripped out. I am permanently winded. I just can't breathe. My respiratory system is paralysed. The drum in the ear nearest to the explosion bursts.

The heat is incredible. I cannot breathe but I am leopard-crawling away from it, scrambling, desperate to get out of it. I make about ten feet, but my energy goes, defeats my urgency to escape. I can go no further. I collapse. It is so fucking hot but I cannot move except to protect my face and head from it with my smouldering red-raw hands. I realise I am deaf from the blast and that my ears are no longer there. Then I realise that my eyelids have been burned too and possibly my eyes. I can barely see. All of me is burned. All of me. Heavy third-degree.

The inferno is no more than the length of a double-decker bus away, the flames are still raging 50 feet high. But I can do no more.

And now the pain comes for me. My God, the pain, Holy Mary, mother of God, Jesus H. Christ. It is useless trying to describe it. From head to toe, every nerve ending in my body is screaming. I am a high-level patrol medic. I know trauma. The adrenaline has run out. I know what a body can take. No one on the planet at that moment is suffering worse pain than me. The skin on my body has gone, a lot of muscle and sinew and tissue too, I have no ears, no hair, my face is torched and caved in, my eye socket and nose are shattered, my collarbone ripped away, my insides torn to shreds. I am so fucking dying. I am dying as hideously as a man can die.

And I am still conscious. My brain is functioning at full capacity. I am so goddam fit, my body and mind won't give out. Give me a gun. Please someone give me a gun. I will give you all I own for a gun. I am on my knees now, my face turned skywards and I am roaring, pleading. *What have I done? What have I done?* It is the pain, but also rage. Tears are pouring down my blistered face, salt in the wounds. I could fight off ten men with this anger, kill them all with my fists and feet.

I am banging through the stages of grief in super-quick time because there's not much time left. Seconds, minutes maybe. My time is up. Violent anger becomes crushing despair. My soul is shattered, I'm head down now and I am sobbing and sobbing. Then another switch, just as rapid, and it's resignation, acceptance of this horrific fate. I am about to die the worst of deaths. It's over.

The hysteria abates and I become rational. I sit down on my arse – at least I still have my arse and cock. No agony there. That's all I'll be taking with me. A bone-skinny arse and a fully functioning dick. The inferno is dying down – it's just a big black and orange fire now. I unlace my molten, smouldering shoes and take them off, placing them side by side. I am on a journey now. Travel light. I don't need shoes where I'm going. I peel away what's left of my socks from what's left of my skin, fold them with my blistered fingers and place them inside the shoes. Neat and tidy, right to the end. Not much of an epitaph but I can't help myself. Always seeking order in my life. Getting my kit right.

I lie back, pull my knees up and together, and I cross my hands over my flayed chest. The pain in my abdomen is off the scale – something has been torn up or out – but I have no scream left in me. I can feel the heat of the hottest time of day but I am getting very cold and I am becoming weak, the fluids running out on me. I am fading to my death. I recognise deep systemic shock, and I like it. I am whispering then I'm silent. I am staring at the sky and the sun is so bright I can't see it. No, it's because I am blind. All I'm getting is light. Or is it the great light you see when you die?

American voices, one on either side. 'Help's on its way, buddy, you hang in there, buddy, we're with you, buddy, we're staying with you, buddy, don't let go, buddy, you're going to make it, buddy ...'

I am grateful for their kindness, just their company. I am groaning and sobbing my words, giving them a running commentary on my slide towards death. 'Fucking hell, fucking hell, oh my God, help me, help me, the pain, I'm going now, I'm dying ...'

The American guys are talking straight over me. They won't give up. Bless them. I can hear and feel their terror and pity. I must be a horrifying sight. There is the tiniest bit of life left in me.

The image won't go away – I am a mouse on a thread suspended from the heavens. It's my last connection to this world. I am swaying on it.

Five minutes, ten, fifteen … I am still here, still hanging by that thread, a little tiny mouse swinging on a gossamer web spool. The Americans are still in my ear, over and over, sounds like they're crying too. 'Hang in there, buddy, you're gonna do it, buddy, you can do this, buddy …' I love them for bigging me up, desperate for me to live. The kindness of strangers, Good Samaritans. Fucking love Americans. They've got heart.

I hear sirens, finally, a long way away. Or is it because my hearing has almost gone and they are right here? No, they're getting louder and there's a lot of them. They're right here. The sirens go off. Doors slam, voices shout, radios fizz and crackle.

'Okay, buddy, they're here now … stay in there, buddy, you're gonna make it, buddy, you're a brave guy, buddy, you can do it, buddy …'

'Thank you, thank you.' Those guys really meant it.

Ah, that's better. Someone has hit me with the good stuff. I am blind and there are already ten million needles in me so I can't tell. But it's a morphine syrette, the medic in me is figuring, because it's washing through me and it's lovely, exactly what I'd have done to the patient on the battlefield. I am still screwed but, fuck me, that's a whole lot better. I am one happy little mouse swinging away.

They're moving fast now. I am on a stretcher and they are running. I can hear the whop-whop-whop of rotor blades. Then the downwash. The churning air is refreshing. I am almost deaf but the roar of the blades and the engine is huge. They place me inside, the noise is squeezed out by the sliding door. Immediate lift-off, not straight up, but banking sharply and accelerating, rocking in the crosswind.

'My name is Doctor Lopez. We are taking you to Orlando Regional, get you some real help. I need you to ask you a few questions. What's your name?'

'James Hull.'

'Nationality?'

'British'

'Home address?'

'Leighton Buzzard, Bedfordshire, UK.'

'Your address here?'

'Pine Court, Pine Trails.'

'Street number?'

'No fucking idea.'

'Occupation?'

'Special Forces Operative.'

'Do you have a health insurance policy?'

'Of course I have fucking insurance, you fucking idiot.'

The morphine is wearing off. I am ashamed of swearing at him. I get that's what they do in the States – ask you a bunch of dumb questions when your head's hanging off and your legs have gone and your stomach's been ripped out – and I get too that part of it is he just wants to keep me talking, keep me conscious.

He gets me too and slips me some morphine and the warm fuzzy feeling comes back. I am in and out of consciousness, back and forth over the border between life and death. He is gently slapping my cheeks, talking, talking, asking me questions about my life, about the accident, about anything that comes into his sweet dumb fucking head ...

'And we're going to do everything for you, James ... You're going to get the best treatment in the world ... you're going to be in great hands ... second to none ... you've made it this far, you're going to make it the whole way ... I promise you that ... just stay with me, James ... they're going to fix you up good as new ...'

I don't give a shit, I just want to die. Sure, I am a tiny bit warm and fuzzy, but I don't want them to keep me alive. It's not worth living any longer, people wiping my arse, feeding me baby food with a rubber spoon, changing the telly channel for me, rest of the world getting on with it.

Wheels hit the helipad – I assume we're on the roof of a building anyhow – doors open, downwash swirling inside, engine whining down, rotors grow quieter, wind dropping, lots of voices and I'm being wheeled like I'm in a race with other stretcher victims on trolleys. The air is freezing now. We are going down in an elevator. Bing! And I'm being sped down another corridor. They are working on me, putting fluid tubes in me, me thinking, *Don't bother, mate. Save it for the guy who's going to make it.*

I am stationary now and I am aware of many people around me. They're all over me. These are critical moments. I am a medic. I get that. But what a waste of time. You're doing what you're trained to do. You can't just walk out and leave me. That's dereliction. But really, *Do yourselves a favour and fuck off home, will you?* Am I saying that, or shouting it? Or just thinking it? Dunno. Don't care. *Pump me with the rest of that morphine then just fuck off, the lot of you. I am a medic too. Come on, look at me, you dickheads. Guy off the street could tell you I'm fucked!*

'James, we are the trauma team. My name is Doctor Howard Smith and I am your lead consultant. I need to ask you some questions.'

'What is this – a fucking job interview? Fuck off with your forms and questions!'

'James, we want to help you. We're going to help you, but I need some basic inf—'

'JUST PUT ME OUT OF THIS FUCKING AGONY, YOU WANKER! I DON'T WANT TO LIVE!'

And the bright lights go out. The thread snaps.

Part 2

2

It was Sunday evening – about 10.30 UK time – and Jamie's mother was in her big armchair in her terraced house in Leighton Buzzard. It had been another cold, showery day, and the chirpy weather forecaster was telling her it had been one of the coldest Augusts on record and the outlook wasn't great. She was in her thick dressing gown and furry slippers and, yes, he was right, it was bloody miserable out there. She grabbed the remote and zapped him into a small dot on the giant screen. There had been no alert, but all the same she picked up her mobile and checked. No, still nothing.

Jamie had texted earlier to say he was going to call after his day's flying. He was going on operational deployment not long after he was back – his first time in a combat zone and she wanted as much of him as she could get before he flew out. By all accounts, it was hell out there, and you just never knew. He'd probably headed straight out for the evening with his mates at the flight school, she figured. No bother, he'll call tomorrow, she was sure. He was a good lad, always did what he promised.

She plugged in the phone, made her way up the stairs and said her prayers. She read for a few minutes but her eyelids began to sink and she reached for the table light. Just as she turned it off, the phone rang downstairs – the house phone – and she leaped up, dashed downstairs, running to it before the answering machine kicked in.

'Hi, love!'

There was quite a long pause, then the voice of an American woman said, 'Am I speaking with Shirley Kristensen?'

'Aye, that'll be me.'

Shirley was thinking cold caller trying to sell her insurance or new windows and she was about to hang up when the voice said:

'It's your son, Miss Kristensen. Jamie. We've got him here in the Orlando Regional Medical Center.'

The caller had a lovely soothing voice but it was no balm for the slashing blow of those words.

'Go on.'

'He's been involved in a flying accident and ...'

'What's happened? What's happened? Is he okay? Can I speak with him?'

Another pause.

'He's alive but he's not okay, Shirley. May I call you Shirley?'

'You can call me what the hell you like, just tell me he's not going to die.'

Another pause.

'It's critical, Shirley, but he's hanging on.'

'NOOOOOO!' Shirley shouted.

Another pause.

'Get on the first flight you can.'

'I will! I will! Orlando – where?'

'Orlando Regional Medical Center. There'll be someone to meet you at Orlando International ...'

'Of course, of course, I'll be there as soon as—'

'I am sorry, Shirley, but I need to tell you this now so you're ready for it ... Jamie's been badly burned. Very badly.'

Shirley's arm fell to her side, the woman's voice still going, 'Shirley? Miss Kristensen? Miss Kristensen, are you still there?'

She replaced the handset, dropped into the armchair, put her head in her hands. *My little boy! My little boy! Be strong, Shirley.*

Be strong for him. For him. Not you. Him. Be strong. Right, pull yourself together ...

She called her neighbour and friend Malcolm and blurted out what had happened. 'Can you help me out with the airfare, Malcolm? I'll pay you back.'

'Of course, I'll be right around.' And he was. It seemed like seconds but there he was, on the doorbell already. He gave her a tight squeeze.

She rang her ex-husband Mick but he wasn't answering so she tried his parents up the road.

Philip, the ex-father-in-law, was asking, 'What do you want him for?'

She explained.

Twenty minutes later, Mick was at the door. They hadn't spoken for months. They didn't speak unless they had to, but she didn't care about that right now. He was Jamie's dad and he had every much of a right to see him as she did. He loved him too. He was theirs.

Next, she called Ryan and Kimberley, Jamie's brother and sister. They were quick on the scene too. Malcolm was on the phone organising flights. They all told her to get her head down and get some sleep. Sleep when her son is 4,000 miles away, battling for his life? They didn't try and tell her again.

Ryan took Shirley and Mick to Heathrow first thing. It was a lunchtime flight but they were at the airport with hours to spare. Shirley was not missing that flight. And, it was ridiculous, but she wanted to be that tiny bit closer to her son and his suffering.

Mick was good. Very quiet and gentle, deep in his own thoughts. But she wanted to be by herself, alone with her prayers, and she found a seat under a flight of stairs. She did not move for two hours, just hugged her thick bible to her chest. She prayed hard – real prayers, the official ones, plus some of her own. She pleaded with the God she had worshipped since the day she took herself to church aged eight, wearing her double-breasted camel coat bought by her mother so she didn't let the family down.

It was late afternoon, Florida time, when they touched down in Orlando. Two officials from the British Consulate greeted them just inside the terminal. Shirley was impressed by this, flattered almost, and then, almost instantly, she was very alarmed. The thought struck her like lightning – these are the people they send when there has been a death. But no, they said, they were there to rush them through customs. Their bags were waiting on the other side. How do they do that, dig out their bags from the hold so fast?

They were hurried through a side door, the diplomats flashing clearance. Shirley was now thinking, *Jamie may not be quite dead yet but he must be very poorly. They want his parents to see him before they shut down the machines. That's what's going on. That's why it's all so slick.*

In the arrivals area, they were introduced to two students from the flight school, one Irish, one English, both sheepish, pale. Apparently, they lived with Jamie in the flight school's courtesy house. They shook hands but Shirley did not take in their names. It was just a few minutes since the aircraft had docked, but they were at the cab rank now. The heat, wet heat, was stifling. The consulate people, solemn and soft-spoken, wished them all the best. Shirley, Mick and the students climbed into the cab, the officials pursed their lips and nodded farewell, and they slipped on to the freeway, a fast-flowing river of traffic.

It took about 20 minutes to reach Orlando Regional in the centre of town. The hospital is huge, covering enough acreage to swallow Leighton Buzzard town centre and more. Dropped at the entrance to the trauma centre, the two students followed them into the elevator to the third floor where the Burns Unit is located. No one spoke. The doors sprung open and the students left them to go through to the unit, parking themselves in a row of seats against the wall.

The hospital was like a luxury hotel, all shining marble, not a speck of dirt, making Luton & Dunstable look like a field hospital. A Father Christmas lookalike – kindly face and white beard – escorted them down the corridor to the changing area outside the trauma unit. Shirley's heart was hammering and she felt faint. She put on a pale blue gown, a hat, surgical gloves and rubber galoshes over her shoes. She disinfected her hands at the dispenser and put on the gloves, Mick the same.

The automatic door opened and – squeak, squeak, squeak – her galoshes carried her down the mirror-clean corridor to the nurses' station. The only other noise was the beeping of monitoring equipment. She kept her head down, not looking through the glass doors into the patients' rooms, clutching her bible to her chest, talking to herself, telling herself to have faith, be strong. She hadn't let go of the bible since she left Leighton Buzzard. Nurses and doctors were gathered around the station. Their faces were grave and they were whispering urgently. She was not aware of Mick now but he must have been at her side.

She introduced herself and they all nodded and blinked and mumbled greetings and shuffled their feet and tried to smile and frown all at once. They carried the look of people who know you are suffering, know you are about to receive a terrible shock. It was hard for them to know what attitude to strike – upbeat and full of hope, or downcast and sympathetic.

One of them, a very pretty girl, stepped forward, shook Shirley's hand firmly and said, 'Miss Kristensen, my name is Renee. I am Jamie's lead nurse. I have put him right in front of the station so we can monitor him twenty-four seven. There he is, right behind you. Room Ten.'

She seemed bold, frank. Kind but tough. Shirley liked her at once. She turned around slowly and stepped towards the glass door. The figure in the bed was enormous – a real-life Michelin Man. The entire body was bandaged except for the head and face, which were covered with some sort of mask or hood. One tube ran from the throat into a machine, another from the nostrils, and at least half-a-dozen other tubes and wires dangled from the body, linked to a bank of machinery. Michelin Man crossed with Frankenstein's monster. *That's not Jamie in those bandages, that's a twenty-stone man, maybe more.*

Shirley turned to the nurses and said, 'My Jamie is a whippet of a lad. He's in the Special Forces. He's as fit as anyone in the UK. There's not an ounce of fat on him. That can't be him.'

A doctor stepped forward, tall and Scandinavian-looking, and introduced himself.

'Miss Kristensen—'

'Shirley, please.'

'Shirley, we have just been discussing the swelling. It's normal for a body to swell after it has been severely burned. That's just the body hanging on to all the fluid it can but ...'

He turned towards the bloated mound of bandages in the bed. He sighed then added, 'But that's not normal, the kidneys are not doing their job. We have made four incisions, a quadrant, in Jamie's upper body. Normally that would relieve the swelling. But, in fact, he has continued to expand and that's ...'

'So, what now? What are you going to do?'

'We need your permission to perform an emergency laparotomy.'

'A what? What's that?'

'We cut him from sternum to bladder, open him right up so we can see everything going on in there. It's the fastest, most reliable way of determining the cause of the problem. The only way.'

'Is it a high-risk operation?'

'Yes, it is. He has already suffered epic trauma, and this is a big procedure which will add significant pressure to the body. But leaving him to swell is an even higher risk. Something abnormal is causing this acute swelling and we need—'

'Fine, fine, fine. You have my full permission. Do whatever you have to do to save my son.'

'We need to find out its cause. Fast. We must operate now.'

He turned to the cluster of medics at the station, clicked his fingers and stabbed a finger towards Room Ten. There was a storm of activity. Two nurses darted towards Jamie's room. One punched the electronic entrance button, the door slid open and the noise of the machines, humming and beeping, flowed into the corridor. Two others were shooting down the far end of the unit, another had seized a phone and was banging numbers.

Shirley walked into Room Ten, stopped and, slowly, made her way over to the bedside. She was trying to believe it, to admit the truth, that it was him, Jamie, her firstborn, that little baby she used to rock in my arms like it was only yesterday. But with all the imagination and will in the world she could not accept that the grotesquely distended heap beneath all that bandage was her son. It was barely recognisable as a human body. She stepped closer and peered down. The ears had all but gone, only dabs of flesh remained. The face and scalp had been smeared in a thick layer of lubricant or emollient, like Vaseline, and wrapped in a see-through mask, like clingfilm or a freezer bag. The skin was red-raw and one of his eye-sockets was caved in. Her hand was quivering a little as she reached for the medical bracelet on his bandaged wrist and rotated it a little. It had a long number on it, some barcodes, just like a supermarket product, and the patient details: Jamie Hull DOB: 7/7/75. Age: 32 Sex: M.

The bible shook against her chest and she clamped her lips, her face and stomach muscles, holding on to her tears for dear life. She moved to seize him in her arms, to put her head on his chest and sob her broken heart out. But she didn't, she couldn't. She didn't dare touch him, the bandages.

She was not aware of Mick or the nurses until she felt a hand on her arm and a voice said, 'Jamie is going to theatre now. Why don't I arrange for someone to direct you to your accommodation? Hubbard House – it's lovely. You can come and see him first thing tomorrow morning. When it's over.'

She walked backwards out of the room, not taking her eyes off him, bible clamped against her under crossed arms. She waited by the nurses' station, aware that she had bitten her lip so hard she had drawn a little blood. An orderly joined the medics in Jamie's room, all gathering around his bed and the wheeled monitors. The doctor checked the reading on a machine, gave the signal and out they rushed, pushing Jamie and his train of equipment. They turned and headed down the corridor like a bobsleigh team at the start of a run. Head down, blood in her mouth, Shirley squeaked her way back down the corridor to the scrubs room. Still, she would not cry.

3

Abdominal compartment syndrome (ACS) occurs when fluid accumulates in such large volumes that the wall of the abdomen can stretch no further. It is quite literally at bursting point, like a balloon filled slowly with water. Once there is no more give in the wall, the pressure on the body rises precipitously. The problem will not fix itself. Drugs are no use. Death is a certainty. The solution is a knife, quickly applied, because under the intensifying pressure, blood flow is reduced and the cardiovascular, pulmonary, renal and gastro-intestinal systems are wrung harder and harder. There is huge stress on the circulation system, the arteries and capillary network are tightly compressed, blood pressure is driven up and up, blockages inevitable. Eventually, and it doesn't take long, the body has no option but to surrender and kill off its host, the organs shutting down like lights going out in a house – 'multiple organ failure' is how the doctor will describe it to you in the waiting room but it will be the cardiac arrest that delivers the death blow. The mortality rate associated with ACS is between 60 and 70 per cent. Hence the rush to get Jamie Hull down that corridor and into the elevator to the theatre. His body already hanging on by the last threads of resistance, his chances of coming back up were very slim.

Down there, he underwent what they call surgical decompression by emergency laparotomy. Crudely, they sliced and peeled him open. And it is crude – because the surgical team are way past medical niceties and tinkering. They have reached the very last resort.

Shirley was back in Room Ten first thing, still dark out. It was as if someone had pricked the Michelin Man with a balloon. He was still hideously bloated, but he was half the size he was the night before. She rested a hand on his bandaged arm, so lightly it was barely touching. There was a shelf above his bed and she placed her bible there so that it was right over his head. Jamie was not devout – he had tried, it hadn't worked for him – but what the hell, he needed every bit of help he can get.

The electronic door whooshed open and the doctor, the Scandinavian-looking one, came in. He was wearing a kind but serious face, head down a little. Doctors don't need to talk to tell you the prognosis. It's written on their faces and in their body language.

'Morning, Shirley, that sure is one tough, resilient boy you have brought into the world.'

'What did you find?'

'It was great you arrived when you did, and great we got him into theatre. We found a badly ruptured colon, which was leaking lethal contaminants, and a badly lacerated liver, which was haemorrhaging. Both life-threatening conditions. He must have hit the ground very hard to cause that level of internal damage.'

He explained how the surgical team cauterised the liver back together, repaired the rip in the colon and cleaned out the spilled faeces as best they could to stop the toxins being absorbed. A ruptured colon is a medical emergency in its own right. The danger is sepsis – bacteria and toxins in the blood – and it will kill you very fast. They had put him on powerful antibiotics, delivered intravenously straight into the bloodstream by an infusion pump. They fitted a catheter for passing urine and a stoma for passing stool. If a ruptured colon was Jamie's only problem, he would still have been blue-lighted into Emergency at breakneck speed. But it was pretty much the least of his problems.

Shirley stared at the heap of bandages, tubes and wires hanging out of every part of it, all trailing into a horseshoe community of bleeping and flashing machines. Forty-eight hours earlier, Jamie could have run up a mountain without pausing for rest; he could have run back-to-back marathons. You could have dropped him in the heart of a desert, a jungle, a swamp or Arctic tundra and he'd have worked his way out, no bother. Now, he couldn't breathe by himself, eat by himself, shit, piss, talk or, in an induced coma, even think or feel. Thank God he couldn't think or feel.

Shirley turned back to the doctor. 'What else? What other injuries?'

'There is a standard system we use to calculate the surface area of the body that has been burned. In Jamie's case, it was easier to calculate that by what hadn't. He has sixty-two per cent full-thickness, third-degree burns, right down to the bone on his lower legs – incredible he managed to keep his feet on those rudder pedals. His legs below the knee are particularly worrisome and we are going to have to make a call on them.'

You'll take my sons legs off over my dead body. That's what Shirley was thinking, firing him a warning look.

'The right side of his body took one hell of a blast – apparently he jumped off the wing – and, as we can see, his face and scalp are also badly burned.'

Shirley looked down at the jellyfish mask covering a face that was barely recognisable as belonging to a human, let alone her handsome son.

'Also, multiple soft-tissue lacerations. The face must have taken a great deal of the impact when he hit the ground. He has suffered a bilateral nasal fracture – that is, his nose is badly broken and that will need some work on it. The bone around his eye has been shattered. That's called a super-orbital left-eye socket fracture. His left index finger is fractured and hyperextended and he has dislocated his collar bone.'

'So apart from that he's right as rain.'

The doctor flashed her an admiring smile. 'You're going to need that famous English sense of humour over the coming days. Jamie's body has taken about as much trauma as a body can take.'

'I'm Scottish.'

'Even better – because you need fighting spirit in a battle.'

Shirley shot him a look. 'So, what are his chances then?'

The doctor looked down at the floor, then pursed his lips and gave her his most sympathetic look.

'He is a remarkable man, your son, Shirley. The fact that he is still with us is a miracle in itself. When they brought him in, we gave him precisely zero chance of survival. These are up there with the worst collection of injuries I have seen on a living being. Most people don't survive third-degree burns to more than about forty per cent of the body – not to mention all his other injuries on top of that. We have had to let go other patients suffering lesser trauma.'

'So what are the odds of survival, his chances now?'

'I'm not going to lie to you, Shirley, raise false hopes. He's hanging on by a very thin thread and he has the fight of his life on his hands.'

'Can you put a figure on it?'

'Anyone else – still close to zero. Jamie – you can tell from his muscle structure he's as fit and strong as they come. He never lost consciousness – that's some resilience. If anyone can make it, he can.'

'So what – twenty to thirty per cent?'

He screwed up his face and rocked his head.

'Fifteen? … Ten?'

He repeated the gurning, not looking her in the eye.

'I've got to be straight with you, Shirley. Five, Shirley. Five, max. I'm sorry.'

There was a pause.

'And what about his quality of life – if he survives?'

'Let's cross that bridge when we come to it.'

4

Bleep, silence, bleep, silence, bleep, silence … hour after hour …
Bleep – the only noise in the room. The window was sealed tight,
aircon refrigerator cold. Shirley was in the armchair next to his
bed. He was motionless. Not so much as a twitch or a groan. Not
even a breath – the ventilator was doing that for him – and bandages so deep she could make out no rise or fall of his chest. If
there was any life under that pile, it sure wasn't showing.

Nurses and doctors came and went, checking monitors and
tubes – the fluids for his electrolytes, the IV antibiotics for the
infections desperate to get at him, the tube to his throat for his
breathing, the naso-gastric tube into the nostrils for his nutrition,
the catheter for his urine, the stoma for his stool, the monitors for
his heart rate and blood pressure, the two tubes draining the fluid
from the pleural cavity in his chest, the VAC suction pump on
his abdomen for sucking out the pus from his guts. They didn't
stitch him up after the laparotomy while there remained a risk of
bloating that would tear open the sutures. And then there was the
everyday risk of an incisional hernia. That's when the intestines
become strangulated and lose their blood supply. If that were to
happen, the medical team could add another emergency injury
to the extensive list already on the clipboard at the foot of his bed.

Bleep, bleep, bleep … Mick came and went. Time blurred.
Shirley was lost in thought and prayer, suspended in a new dimension. Every few minutes, she'd lean forward to look at her son. It
was a shock every time. She took in a sharp intake of breath or

covered her mouth or shook her head, the unspilled tears stinging her eyes (she was determined to stay strong for him). It never
got easier looking at a face that she couldn't recognise as her son's.
The surgeons had told her they had no plans to work on the face
for weeks or months partly for fear of it becoming infected and
partly because his body was under quite enough stress. There was
no harm in waiting.

Every inch of the face – and most of the scalp – had been
scorched in the flames and most of it was further damaged when
he jumped and slammed into the earth. The face, and the right
shoulder, took the impact from 20 feet. 'Self-amputated' was the
ugly phrase one of the doctors used for the mangled stubs of his
ears. Like the ears had made a conscious choice to chop themselves off.

With the nose and one eye socket crushed, both eyes appeared
to have sunk. The delicate eyelids were easy prey for the flames,
and the eyebrows too had been incinerated, along with all but a
few tufts of the hair on his head. The eyes seemed twice as big as
normal and, unable to blink, they stared blankly at the ceiling.
Jamie was an extremely handsome young man – a real hit with
the girls – but his injuries had transformed him into a creature
more closely resembling a prehistoric fish under a glass case in
a natural history museum, an impression compounded by the
slimy gel and see-through mask. Moreover, owing to the peculiar nature of the injuries to the cavities and his cheeks, plus the
destruction of his hair and eyebrows, the eyes appeared not only
to have sunk into the skull but also to have slid an inch or so
down the face.

Shirley yearned to hug him but she still couldn't. So she spoke
to him. All the time. She'd say anything. Just connect, hope some
of it would be registering deep in his stupefied mind, just as it
does with a baby in the womb. *Be strong, Jamie, be strong … Don't*

flatline on me, my love ... we'll get you home ... this hospital's incredible, like a five-star hotel, you're in the best hands ... I'm not going home till your ready ... when you're a bit better I'll take you into the roof garden just outside, it's beautiful ... they do a lovely cappuccino in the café ... Any old nonsense.

Throughout the day the medics gathered and dispersed at the nurses' station, like they were in a time-lapse clip, masks around their necks, leafing over clipboards, glancing in at Jamie, rushing left and right, patients on gurneys sliding past, fast one way, slow the other, the frame of the glass door giving the impression she was watching television with the mute button on, that none of this was real, the soundtrack in loop mode ... *bleep, bleep, bleep.* Each bleep another second of life, of recovery, his body putting in the shift of all shifts to get itself back to normal.

In the afternoon, Renee, the nurse she really liked, was back on duty and the door whooshed open for her. She strode in, radiating energy, purpose, kindness. Jamie's angel. That's the way Shirley saw it, felt it, the aura of her. There was something about her. She held the key. That wasn't crazy God stuff. It was a mother's intuition. She knew Renee was going to give herself to him. When the chopper landed on the roof and the trauma team were waiting for him, it was Renee who challenged the team and said, 'Come on, let's give him a chance. We fight for him.' The others were not so sure. No one gave him any hope. They had seen admissions with half these burns go to the wall in no time, the sliding wall down in that refrigerated morgue in the basement. Renee was the one who pushed for him. Least, that's what she said and Shirley had no reason to be doubt her.

Shirley watched her fussing around him, like he was her own child. She was talking to him as though he were sitting up fully alert, in her beautiful Southern Belle accent, as soothing on the ear as the cooling emollient on his skin. Shirley realised she was smiling for the first time since she took the call back home.

Renee finished her inspection of the equipment and spun around, a big smile revealing a perfect pair of teeth. My, she was pretty. Jamie would like her. She was his type. Athletic, positive, tough, kind, competent – and a strawberry blonde too. He loved strawberry blondes. His beautiful on-off Canadian girlfriend Terri was a strawberry blonde. That was a thought – how was she going to tell Terri? How would Terri react if she was to visit him in this state?

'Okay, Shirley, we have to dress Jamie's wounds and change his bandages. Why don't you get yourself a coffee – or sit out on the terraced garden? Come back when we're done.'

'I know, it's beautiful, very calming, but may I stay, please?'

Renee tilted her head and screwed up her face. 'You sure?'

'I can handle it.'

'Great, then let's get to work. I'll get the other nurse.'

Shirley helped the nurses rock Jamie back and forth as they peeled off the layers of bandage and dressing. Renee was right. It was an appalling sight, swathes of charred flesh deep into the tissue. Only the groin area, the rear of the upper legs and his back from the shoulder blades down had escaped the inferno. The plastic surgeons, Dr Gupta and Dr Simmian, had wasted no time in getting to work. They had performed multiple escharotomies on his entire right side – shoulder, arm, chest and lower right leg. This was the side that had taken the furious blast of flame when he stood on the wing. The left would be next, soon.

A full-thickness or third-degree burn means the top three layers – the epidermis, the dermis and the hypodermis (subcutaneous tissue) – have been destroyed. The eschar is the leathery crust, the shrivelled, dead tissue, that has formed. An escharotomy is the procedure by which a deep surgical incision is made in the affected area in order to loosen the constriction, reduce the pull on what's left of the tissue. The sooner it's performed the better the final outcome. It is not a life-saving procedure, it's a life-enhancing one – should the patient survive. To Shirley, Jamie's arm and leg looked like split sausages, his torso like a joint of scarred pork that had left too long under a too-hot grill.

The hands had been the first to get the treatment from the plastic surgeons. That was standard procedure. They had been very badly damaged, especially the back of them, when he was battling to bring in the aircraft, his left hand on the control stick, his right on the throttle. The surgeons make the hands a priority for good reason. We need our hands for the majority of the important tasks in our daily lives: eating, dressing, washing, brushing teeth, driving, writing, typing, operating a telephone, playing sports … If the elasticity goes, life becomes immeasurably more difficult, the patient more dependent on the help of others, his activities limited. If they leave the hands untreated, the skin and tissue stiffen and knot, webbing the fingers, turning the hands into useless flippers. Sort the hands and the patient has a fighting chance of fending for themselves. And the insurance companies like that too. Imagine the cost of all those carers over a lifetime!

Representatives of the insurance company were all over the hospital from the moment they were informed. The dials of the cab meter were already spinning wildly and the underwriters were sweating. The cost of the care Jamie had received in the first 48 hours was already over a quarter of a million dollars and the bill was rising fast. In all, the emergency treatment alone was going to run to millions.

Before flying out to Orlando, Jamie had gone into the small market town of Tring to take out cover for the unlikely event of him suffering an accident at the flying school. He hated taking out insurance for his travels. Not once in all his many trips overseas had he ever made a claim. He bridled and moaned a little at the £93.45 the little High Street outfit charged him.

'Hundred quid, give or take – that's a bit steep, isn't it? Is that your best offer?'

It was turning out to be the best £93.45 a man could ever spend.

5

In the blasting heat of the cockpit, his body wrapped in flame, it was strength of character and inner cool that had saved Jamie from losing control, going into a spin and piling in. Or fleeing the pain, bailing out at 500 feet and plunging to his death. He was on fire but he stayed put, sitting in the flames, working the controls, bringing the plane in, going through the emergency landing protocol just as he had been taught. Out on the wing, he had even had the cool to wait a couple of seconds, his right side blowtorched by the mini-firestorm, until the stricken plane was low enough for him to leap.

His mind and spirit had done their bit. Howling in the long grass of the airfield, the baton of survival was handed over to his body, a body in supreme condition, the only type with a chance of withstanding the savagery of such an assault. It wasn't a task for the mind or the spirit. There was nothing to be cool or strong about. He was just rolling around on fire – and that doesn't take any skill or knowledge or inner resolve. He was behaving as any mammal would. It was down to his body whether he could hang on or not, not up to him.

It was the hypothermia, the shock from the blood and fluid loss, that threatened to get him. His inner body functions were already undergoing radical upheaval. Massive redistribution of body fluid was underway. Within 20 to 30 minutes the water content in his burns would shoot up by 80 per cent. That fluid has to come from somewhere and, without a fresh source from outside, the water has to be drawn from within, depleting the resources for his organs to near nothing. In that fluid, his electrolytes, so vital for the body to carry out its functions, were ebbing to nothing. And his body was devouring all its protein. He needed a bunch of tubes in him. Fast. Not to mention a massive shot of opiates to knock him into next week.

The minutes had ticked by, Jamie conscious throughout, the distant drone of the helicopter growing a little louder until it was thundering overhead in the hover, flattening the grass. The paramedics had leaped from the open door into the sprint, thrown themselves on their knees and gone straight to work on him. Another minute or so, it would have been all over. Then, the crew could have taken as long as they wished to deal with the situation, zip him up and load him aboard – or maybe leave it to a road ambulance to deal with the removal, and upwards and onwards they'd go to the next crisis, or back to the helipad, waiting for the next 911 scramble.

Between his body, mind and soul, Jamie had done everything a man could to keep alive. The first responders had done their bit too. Now it was over to the medics from Orlando Regional Medical Center.

The treatment of major burns is a tremendous challenge for a medical team, involving round-the-clock attention and specialists from multiple disciplines. Speed is of the essence. Every minute counts right at the start, then every hour over the first few days or so. The patient is hypercritical for the first few weeks, then just plain critical for the months that follow.

Even if the immediate battle for physical survival is won, it is just the first, the quickest and most intense in a long war, a gruelling campaign to put the body back in order, to stop the mind and spirit from collapsing under the attritional physical stress, the dread of a fucked-up body, the dread of looking into a mirror, of a fucked-up life, of being helpless and dependent on others to get by.

The fight goes on for years, forever – unless you are a saint, an extreme sado-masochist or a madman. No one bounces back from severe burns. They crawl back, inch by inch. If you want to inflict the worst kind of torture on your enemy then torch him to a cinder, leave his life hanging in the wind by a gossamer thread. Then sit back laughing and watch him battle, hour after hour, day after day, year after year, to restore his body, his spirit, his life – restore each of them to some sort of semblance of their former selves. That is what Fate had done to Jamie Hull.

Go on, let's see what you've got, Jamie lad. Think you're hard? Think you've got your life sorted now, eh? Well, come back from this, tough guy. Thought you were going on operational deployment with Britain's elite regiment, huh? Maybe you should have stayed in Leighton Buzzard, become a professional villain, a junkie. This is what happens if you get above your station in life. You get hurled back down in flames.

And for an extra challenge, extra laughs, Fate had layered on an emergency laparotomy to the immense burden already on the body, plus a shredded colon, a split liver and some shattered bones. He'd made it into a second day, but only just, by the skin of a cat's whisker. He was still deep in Hail Mary territory – and it was going to be some time before the Virgin Mother no longer had to field those calls. Most of them from his own mother, sitting there right next to him. She was going nowhere and those prayers were going to keep coming.

Once the trauma team had stabilised him, covering the burns was the next imperative. Early wound cover is vital in order to prevent the onset of infection. Multi-resistant organisms need no second invitation to tuck into all that lovely raw flesh. It's party time for the gangs of bacteria lurking in the shadows. Even if heavy security is put in place to bar their entry, they will keep swarming to find a way in. There will always be gate-crashers at a party and they will have zero respect for their host's property. They will trash everything inside.

Jamie's team had done everything they could, as fast as they could, to ward off the intruders but everyone understood that a showdown was brewing. When they force an entry, a mass fight breaks out. Heavy back-up is essential. The mass fight has a name – sepsis – and the back-up to beat it off comes in the form of saturation antibiotics. But sepsis is not the only threat. The fight spreads, it becomes a neighbourhood free-for-all. Renal failure, pneumonia, septicaemia and hypovolemic shock want a piece of the action too. Hell, yeah. Why should they miss out? It's party time.

6

Jamie's father went home at the end of the first week. Mick had to return to work, get back on the road as a long-distance lorry driver, keep the money coming in. He'd stay in touch and fly back to Orlando when he could. His son's life was on pause, but his had to go on. Besides, there was not a whole lot he could do to help. It didn't matter if he was worried and upset at Jamie's bedside or worried and upset in the cab of his HGV. And ex-spouses are 'exes' for a reason – Shirley was unlikely to miss him. Mick had been gentle and quiet all week, as anxious and despondent as Shirley, but she was pleased to be on her own now, to focus on Jamie, no distractions. She was staying a two-minute walk away at Hubbard House, a charity-funded hospitality home for the relatives of the long-term sick, as fine as any hotel she'd ever stayed in.

Like all new residents she had been embraced by the community from the minute she checked in, all of them bonded by tragedy and worry. Hubbard House was the perfect refuge. She had a lovely room with an en-suite bathroom and a small lounge area, a communal living and dining room, three meals a day, full refrigerators for snacks and drinks, and doting, compassionate volunteers on hand 24 hours a day to help with practicalities or offer up a shoulder to cry on.

Jamie's fate was going to hang in the balance for the foreseeable. He was going nowhere for a very long time – at least not in this world. She didn't need one of the doctors to tell her that.

She only had to glance at the bed. His was an entirely artificial existence, a phantom life. The life-support machinery was doing all his living for him. Turn off any one of them and he'd die. Flick a switch, tug out a tube, and he'd be on his way. It was a sprint to death or a marathon to recovery. That's the way Jamie – ever the competitor – would see it. He was in the race of his life, a race for his life.

Shirley was settling into a routine, going through the daily schedule as if in a drug-induced trance. There were some real drugs in her system too. She'd been sleepless for the first two nights since getting the call, stricken with worry, her head spinning with dark thoughts: the pain he must have gone through, the fear of losing him, the tough life ahead if he made it, explaining all that to him when he came around, handing him the mirror. On the third night, exhaustion got the better of her and she as good as passed out on the bed – only for a terrifying nightmare to tear her from her peace.

She wanted to avoid taking her sleeping pills so that she could be sharp to deal with the doctors, make the right decisions for Jamie. But the fog of sleeplessness was fraying her judgement and shredding her already ragged nerves. She dug out the lorazepam, a benzodiazepine prescribed to treat insomnia and anxiety. She was so grateful for the respite from the anguish, the next morning she went straight to the hospital chapel and offered up a prayer of thanks to lorazepam, God-given manna from heaven.

In this new Groundhog Day routine she rose early and, refreshed after a deep sleep and a delicious breakfast, comforted and fortified by a hug with a fellow resident and a volunteer, she made the short walk across the way back to the trauma centre. She went to the waiting room on the third floor, sat down next to the smiling Santa Claus character on reception, and waited to be called through.

She had to sit it out in the waiting room a little longer than normal that morning, staring up at some *Oprah*-style talk show on TV, all the guests shouting at each other and storming off set. Jamie was in theatre undergoing another skin graft, the plastic surgeons working the patches into the body quilt they were making for him. There had been a road accident overnight and some suitable fresh skin had been harvested from the cadaver. Donor skin has to be the right match for the recipient's in thickness, colour and texture. When the skin comes from another person, there is a high chance of the body rejecting it because the immune system detects a foreign invader and attacks it. Ideally, you want an identical twin's skin. But, the sooner they could get any skin down, cover the charred flesh, the better. That's what they kept telling her.

At some point, Jamie's surgical team were going to harvest skin from his own donor sites too, but there wasn't going to be much to work with. Of the 35 per cent of his body surface to escape the flames, some areas were unsuitable for harvesting – the groin, the back of the neck, the palms. Only his back, buttocks and the inner and rear of his thighs offered workable skin. With his body under so much stress as it was, stripping down those sites would have to be done in small stages.

Of greater concern in the moment was the very real threat of sepsis. Whenever an area of skin is grafted from a donor site on the patient's body, there is a high risk of bacterial infection leading to blood poisoning and all manner of complications that flow from that. Sepsis is the body's life-threatening response to infection, when the immune system overreacts and starts to damage tissue and organs. Jamie's body was already at the highest possible level of risk of developing sepsis. Any further increase in that risk and the medics may just as well have injected the poison into his blood and be done with it. It would be a self-defeating exercise to expose an even greater area of Jamie's body to potentially lethal moulds.

So, for the time being, in order to get him covered as quickly as possible, the surgeons were going to be using temporary skin donated by the recently deceased or taken from animals, pigs mostly. They do this when the patient is seriously compromised, buying some time until he regains some strength.

When the patient is his own donor, this is called an autograft and it is the best option for long-term treatment. When the skin is harvested from another human being it is called an allograft. When the donor is a pig or another animal, it is called a xenograft. Jamie was going to need a great many allografts and xenografts because the body rejects the former after about a week to ten days and the latter after three to five days.

The skin is the largest organ in our bodies and its outer layer, the epidermis, is the body's wrapper, its protective packaging, keeping the harmful stuff out. It is our defence system against incoming biological and chemical attacks. The outermost layer of the epidermis is made up of dead cells that shed and turn to dust at a rate of about 20,000 pieces a minute. Ever wondered where all that dust in your house and in your hoover bag comes from? It's your dead skin mostly. Snakes are not the only creatures to shed their skin. The human body is constantly generating fresh cells, giving the body a whole new skin covering every month. Outwardly and imperceptibly, you become a new person 12 times a year.

Below it, lies the dermis. The dermis teems with activity, carrying out a host of functions vital to our survival. There you will find your hair follicles (up to five million of them), your sweat glands (about the same again) and the sebaceous glands (a sort of self-moisturiser to lubricate the skin and hair). There, too, you find blood vessels – the branch lines of the circulation system – and lymphatic vessels, which serve three key roles in our immunity system: delivering white blood cells to fight infection, removing waste matter, draining fluid from our tissues into the blood.

The third layer of skin is the hypodermis, often called the subcutaneous layer, and it sits between the dermis and our tissues and organs. It's where we store our fat and it fastens the whole spread of our skin to the body within, maintaining body temperature by keeping in the heat, and acting as a shock absorber of external blows. Jamie's skin grafts had to be 'full-thickness', meaning he needed all three layers complete with blood and lymphatic vessels, hair follicles, sweat and sebaceous glands.

In short, your skin is not merely a cosmetic attribute that defines your colour and keeps the rain off the important bits. It is a vital organ in its own right. Strip or scorch away 65 per cent of a body's dermis, epidermis and hypodermis, and you're in major trouble. This is why the medical team in Orlando were racing against the clock to give Jamie new skin, a temporary one then a permanent one. He was effectively at the start of an epic, ongoing organ transplant operation. Assuming he hung in there and allowed the plastic surgeons to keep slapping on the new skin, he was looking at two or three years before the transplant was complete. They could worry about trying to make him look pretty again down the line.

When Santa Claus put down the phone from the nurses' station and gave Shirley the green light that morning, telling her Jamie was up from theatre, she hurried over to the changing area outside the Burns Unit and her new routine recommenced. She grabbed a clean gown from the peg, hat and gloves from the boxes and put the galoshes on over her shoes, wrung her hands under the antibacterial dispenser, pressed the buzzer to be admitted and waited for the click of the door. Just like the day before and the day before that, she got the update on his progress at the nurses' station. Or rather, the lack of it because, for the time being, his life was effectively suspended, on hold. He was frozen in time. Progress was not dying.

The door to Room Ten slid open and she went to stand at the head of the bed, looking down at his unrecognisable face below the aspic and the silk veil. She talked to him like he was sitting across the breakfast table from her. She told him about her new friends at Hubbard House, the delicious breaded chicken and coleslaw she'd had for supper, the silly talk show she'd been watching out in the waiting room, news about the visitors heading out from the UK to see him, the oppressive heat …

For the rest of the morning, she settled back in the armchair right next to the bed, the medics silently going about their business on the other side of the glass door, the voices and telephones no more than a muffled hum, the cleaners scrubbing and scouring and spraying, the sharp stench of antibacterial disinfectants filling her nostrils, the slow time marked by the methodical bleep of the machines behind her.

When a specialist consultant on his round made his visit (curiously, all Jamie's principal consultants were male), Shirley would hit him with a barrage of questions. To a man, they were cagey but honest, a couple maybe a little too honest, blunt even. She was definitely on a collision course with one of them – and good luck to him as far as Shirley was concerned. Mostly, though, the consultants were doing a great job in explaining the science, detailing the upcoming procedures, managing her expectations and generally keeping her in the loop and out of the dark.

Of course, they couldn't say for sure if Jamie would make it – she knew that – but it was the question bursting her soul apart at the seams: *Was Jamie going to make it?* She couldn't help it erupting from her mouth each time a man with a little grey on the temples appeared at the bedside. These men were veteran handlers of a thousand worried sick next-of-kins, masters of ambiguity, opacity and bet hedging. With a grave face and the odd flash of a warm smile and the sympathetic nod of a head, patiently each one would set about talking her down from the high perch of her desperate urgency, counselling hope and caution in equal measures. She'd feel very slightly reassured by the calm manner and the big words, but she was absolutely none the wiser when the door whooshed back open and the expert moved on to the next bed.

In between the consultants' rounds, the nurses came and went, in and out, in and out, all day long, checking the machines and tubes, crazy busy but always finding time for Shirley.

So, she learned, this is what they mean by 'round-the-clock' care: non-stop monitoring, scanning the data for fresh trouble, adjusting fluid levels, medication dosages, dressing the wounds, the physios rushing in to bend his limbs and joints for half an hour twice a day, keep those muscles and ligaments from stiffening and hardening beyond repair.

It was the nurses she was getting to know and like the best, the honest, uncomplaining infantry in Jamie's army of medics. She was delighted when, for the third day in a row, the shifts changed over and Renee swept in for the evening stint, full of purpose and superhuman cheer. If any voice was to work its way through the dense fog of barbiturates and make contact with Jamie at some level of consciousness, it was Renee's syrupy Southern drawl.

'So, Jamie honey, how you doin' this evenun'? You're getting a little better every day and it sure won't be long before we've got you fit as a flea and a fiddler once again ... now, you be a honey and let me just turn you a little there, get at that bandage ... that's it, honey, thank you ... now, am gonna tell you a little story cuz you never gonna guess what happened to me last night ...'

She talked just the same with Shirley, aware of her pain and struggle too. Unlike Jamie's, it was the pain and struggle no one can see, only guess at. Shirley was putting on a brave face. She was determined to be strong for her son. Unless someone's sobbing or having hysterics, most people don't clock the grief and anguish of others. But Renee did. She got it.

Halfway through the morning, Renee looked at her watch and turned to Shirley. 'I've got my break now. You want to join me for one of these? I'm trying to quit but, you know, it's stressful sometimes.'

She lifted a packet of cigarettes from her scrubs pocket, discreetly, her back to the glass door, like they were school kids making sure teacher didn't see. Shirley had got the impression that smoking was virtually a crime in the States – you couldn't even smoke in the breezy, wide-open hanging garden – and she liked the friendly conspiracy of it. She'd given up cigarettes way back, but allowed herself the occasional one at times of high stress or high fun.

'Sure, why not?'

The two of them took the staff lift down to the ground floor and lit up in the smoking shelter, Renee puffing furiously so she could get back to work. She was making rapid small talk, like they were old friends, telling her about her home life, what she was doing at the weekend, like everything was normal – her friendly, easy manner creating the happy illusion that Jamie was going to be just fine, of course he was. Owing to the gravity of Jamie's condition, most of the medics tended to give Shirley a look to match, the solemn, respectful look of the undertaker. But not Renee. She radiated a tough optimism that said, *Leave it to me Shirley, I'm gonna will that boy of yours back to life. Now, don't you go worryin' yourself sick about it ...*

When they headed back up, buoyed by Renee's energy, Shirley collected her bag from Jamie's room, bowed her head and said a prayer over him. At the door, she blew him a kiss and said, 'I'll see you first thing in the morning, my love.'

Keeping her eyes on him, she stepped backwards into the passageway and a voice said, 'Whoo, I'm sorry. I almost knocked right into you there ...'

It was Dr Smith, the one who seemed to be in overall charge of Jamie's case. She liked Dr Smith, not least because he was short like her and didn't look down on her when talking but straight at her. He was courteous and gentle too.

'Anyhow, I was just coming to see you. We need to talk about Jamie's legs.'

'What about his legs?'

'Well, it's just what we feared was going to happen. The mould colonising on the lower extremities just keeps coming back, no matter how fast we debride it – I mean scrape it off.'

'But what about all those antibiotics?'

'We have taken a number of samples and there's a lot of mould building up. The primary strain is one called Fusarium, a very aggressive and invasive fungus that causes something called aspergillosis. We have put him on a heavy course of orconazole, an anti-fungal. But, Shirley, Jamie is seriously immunocompromised and—'

'What does all that mean? Forgive me, I didn't go to medical school,' she asked with a smile.

'I'm sorry. Jamie's ability to fight off infection is very limited right now. Any number of these moulds, these fungi, are crying out to set up home on him. There is a very real danger he will develop very serious infection, which will get into his blood and poison him. I'm talking about sepsis and septic shock here. And that can lead to—'

'So, what are you going to do about it?'

Dr Smith puckered his lips and hugged his clipboard a little tighter.

'We're going to take another look at his legs tonight while they're doing a graft, excise some more flesh, a biopsy, see exactly what's going on down there.'

'Then what?'

'Then we'll have a meeting, make a call on it, decide on a plan. But we can't wait too long. We must act. It's not an emergency quite yet but we're not far from that point. It's very urgent.'

'Fine, just keep me posted. I'll be here first thing again. And you know I'm just across the way in Hubbard House if you need to make a call on it the night.'

Her mind turning over, Shirley took a couple of steps down the passageway, swung about and said, 'Doctor Smith?'

He looked over his shoulder. 'Yes, Shirley?'

'What's the most likely course of action?'

She hated it when the doctors looked down at their feet, and that's what he did before looking up and walking back to her.

'Shirley, the consensus right this moment ... we think the safest option, Shirley, is to take off his legs.'

7

It was the next morning and the consultants had finished their meeting.

'Over my dead body you'll take his legs off!'

Shirley hollered it and everyone at the nurses' station stopped what they were doing and looked up.

She took two steps forward and Dr Smith took two steps back.

She continued: 'You may just as well put a bullet in his head as take his legs off. Jamie is a man of action. He doesn't want a life with no legs! He'd rather be dead. I'm telling you.'

Dr Smith held up his hands, like Shirley was holding a shooter or a blade. The other medics frozen to the spot in the passageway and at the station.

'Woah, easy. Okay, okay. I hear you, Shirley. Amputation's not something we consider lightly, you understand. But we're talking about a serious risk of sepsis here. That could kill him.'

'So would losing his legs. Sitting in a wheelchair or hobbling on prosthetics … I'm telling you, he'd take the sepsis every time.'

'Okay, Shirley. We'll have another think, another meeting. We won't do anything without your permission.'

'Damn right you won't.'

Shirley stamped down the passageway and made her way out to the hanging garden. She dropped into a stone bench and crossed her arms, the terraced gardens below like a giant stairway. She really liked Dr Smith – he genuinely listened to her – and she didn't like to talk to him that way. But even if pigs flew under a blue moon through a blizzard in hell they were never going to have those legs of his in the waste bin. If Jamie was conscious, he'd say the same. It was her son, after all. He'd back her up on that. No, there would be no amputations. That was the end of it.

The sound of a passenger jet made her look up. Silhouetted against the clear blue sky, the sun glistening on the fuselage, it was heading straight towards the hospital. Its wheels were down and it was so low they appeared to be brushing the rooftops, the noise of it drowning out the traffic on the avenue below and making the birds flee. Shirley craned her neck further and further back until, whining hysterically, the jumbo jet was right overhead, plunging the garden into shadow. Then it was gone and the peace returned.

There was a tap on her shoulder. It was one of the male nurses.

'Ah, Shirley, there you are. Doctor Gupta and his colleague would like to see you. They're in the conference room back in Burns.'

Dr Gupta stood up as she strode into the room. His kind face was smiling (good sign). They shook hands. Shirley sat down, leaning forward, forearms on the table, looking right at him.

'Shirley – may I call you Shirley?'

'You can call me what you like if you tell me you're not to hack my son's legs off.'

'I think I can save Jamie's legs.'

Shirley sprung from her seat and threw out her arms, like an evangelical preacher.

'You can! Really? You're going to save his legs?'

She clenched her fists and shook the air, like she had just scored a screamer from 30 yards. She was so happy she had to stop herself kissing him.

'This is what I'm proposing to do. It is imperative we get rid of that mould – or reduce it as best we can. It's burrowed down into his muscles and necrotised the tissue, killed most of it. That's bad news. It's working its way into his system. But if I was to cut out the muscles, back and front, he wouldn't be able to walk again so you might just as well take his legs off.'

'So, what then?'

'The mould is worse in the front because it took the full blast of the flame and there's not much left there anyhow. Skin regenerates, muscle doesn't. He's never going to get those muscles back. Science is yet to find a way of creating new muscle or transplanting it from donors. So …'

'So … go on … how?' Shirley was tipping forward on her seat.

'I'm going to excise the muscles out of the front of the shins – excise meaning cut them out right to the bone. We have to get them out fast. The bacteria is rampant, literally eating him, and it won't be long before it spreads deep into the back ones and then it's just a question of when it enters his circulation. The mould on the calves is not quite so bad, just on the skin at the moment, so we'll keep debriding them, scraping it off. I'm going to leave them right where they are.'

'What does that mean? I mean, if he has half his muscles out, how will he function?'

'It means he'll still be able to walk assuming, well …'

'Assuming he makes it. It's okay, you can say that. I know he's going to make it.'

Dr Gupta puckered his lips, looked up and smiled with his eyes, showing his admiration for her spirit.

'He will be able to walk well, even run a little. Not like he used to. He won't be able to play competitive sport and he would fail a medical for the Armed Forces. But he'll be able to go about his daily business. He will lose what's called his dorsal inflection so he will walk a little funny, like he's on the balls off his feet, but it will be as good as imperceptible after a time. Only he will really notice.'

'So, when do you plan to do it?'

'Right away. There's no time to waste. Every second we sit here, the risk of sepsis increases. Do I have your permission? I have to stress to you that this operation is a high risk. There is no guarantee it will save him from a fatal infection in the end. Also, his body is hanging on by a thread as it is, and this will place it under even greater strain. It could even—'

'I understand.' She looked him in the eye.

He lifted his elbows and spun the form he was leaning on 180 degrees, pushing it across the table. Shirley seized the pen, squiggled her signature and pushed it back.

'Doctor Gupta, thank you. If Jamie does live, what you're about to do will save his life in a different way. I know the risks. He'd ask you to do the same, I can assure you.'

He nodded and moved quickly for the door. He thrust his head back in and said, 'Jamie does have insurance, doesn't he?'

Shirley said, 'You know, if one more person asks me that, I'm reaching for the nearest scalpel. Yes, he has bloody insurance.'

8

Dr Gupta hurried away to get scrubbed up and Shirley went to see Jamie before he went down. She had stopped to talk to Renee when Jamie came zooming towards her, propelled by a burly orderly, surrounded by nurses wheeling the life support machinery, a web of tubes and wires hanging over him. She watched them pull the bed into the lift, his veiled head the last of him to disappear. She went into Jamie's room, empty but for the armchair, and took the bible from the shelf. Eyes down, tears stinging, the Good Book squeezed to her chest, she made her way slowly out of the ward and back into the mellow evening heat of her secret garden.

Dr Gupta and the surgical team went straight to work, cutting away all the damaged muscle and the fascia – the sheath of tough fibrous tissue covering the bone. They worked on both Jamie's tibias – the shinbones – from knee to ankle, cutting, scraping and scouring down to the bone. It was the necrosis they were after – all that dead and damaged tissue was a free buffet for the bacteria – but the surgeons could leave nothing on the bone. Everything had to go: every scrap the flames had left of the muscle, the nerves and the arteries. One day he might be able to say he was just skin and bone down there, but when they wheeled him back up a couple of hours later, a couple of plain bones, clean as leeks, were all that remained.

All that high-tech live machinery packed so neat and tight around those limbs, those bundles of muscle, tissue and nerves to which he had never given but a passing thought or glance – the whole lot had had been cleared out, sacrificed for the greater good. If Jamie was still to have a life to lead, it could never be the same as, or even similar to, the one that had gone before. These fascial compartments, as the doctors called them, were non-vital body accessories, peacetime luxuries expendable in a war, weighing down the sinking ship of his body, now jettisoned to keep him afloat a while longer.

Non-vital, in an existential sense – yes. But these unsung body parts had been vital to him in another sense. Without them, he would never have been able to transform his life, convert himself from teenage misfit and potential life-loser into a top, multi-discipline athlete, British Army officer and elite Special Forces operative. They had carried him on countless runs, hikes, army exercises, all manner of sporting contests, over the mountains and bogs of Wales, through the wooded wilderness of remote Norway, the jungles of Central America, the Arctic tundra and the savannahs and deserts of Africa, the swamps of America's Deep South. Now, with a few swipes of a blade and a curette, it was all gone and with it any hope of ever repeating those experiences and resuming the life he loved. If there was a life for him to lead down the line, it was going to be very different from the one he had been living and loving.

Jamie would never walk normally again, let alone complete an assault course or a 30-mile march in full kit. All else being well and he recovered sufficiently to stand up again and succeed in being discharged from hospital, he was now officially, permanently disabled. There were no corrective procedures, no treatments, no hope of natural regeneration to restore the former functioning of his lower extremities.

But, if he was ever to wake up, Shirley was convinced the expensive fare he had paid for his return journey to consciousness was worth every penny. He would wake up and look down to find his legs were still in situ, just as before, the tibia and fibula still attached to the knee and ankle, a pair of feet waiting there for a pair of socks and shoes. He'd understand that they had to throw something overboard.

Shirley looked at her watch, pushed herself up from the pew kneeler, made her way out of the chapel and took the lift back up to the third floor. Santa Claus rang through to the nurses' station and she was given the all clear to scrub up and head straight on in. A new set of whirring machinery had been placed at the foot of his bed, tubes filled with blood and fluids running to his lower legs, disappearing beneath the heavy bandages and connected to bags hung from pegs like clothes on a washing line.

Shirley went to the head and started talking to him, as she always did on coming in, explaining the procedure he had been through, justifying her decision, her pride in fighting to keep his legs, hoping the voice, if not the words themselves, were finding a way through. When she had exhausted all she had to say, she sat down in the armchair and, lulled by the rhythmic bleeping of the life support, quickly fell into a half sleep.

She woke with a start. Dave, one of the nurses, was rushing through the door, his face frozen in alarm. He reached out for one of the blood bags and swore under his breath. He looked at the readings, moving fast along the monitors. Shirley sprung from the chair.

'What's happening?'

Dave ignored her for a moment, his face screwed in thought, absorbed in the machinery. He turned to the wall and slapped the alarm buzzer.

'Screen outside says his blood volume is dropping.'

Dr Gupta and a junior were half running when they reached the glass door. They were there in seconds. Gupta made a quick inspection of the monitors, squeezed a blood bag, turned to Dave and said, 'Order six units of blood – now! Then get those bandages off his legs.' To the assistant, 'We need to cauterise immediately.' To Shirley, 'Please, wait outside.'

She turned for the door and heard Dave slapping the phone receiver back into the wall cradle, whispering, 'Cauterise?'

As the door slid shut she caught snatches of Dr Gupta's reply, ' ... only option ... last resort ... fast.'

She watched the assistant dash down the corridor and disappear into a storeroom, returning moments later at a shuffling run, clutching some equipment. An orderly was coming from the other direction at pace, carrying the see-through blood bags. She watched them unwrap Jamie's legs with rapid, forceful movements, nothing like the gentle unravelling when the nurses dressed his wounds. Dave had pulled up the waste-disposal can, his foot on the pedal to keep the lid up, and they tossed in the bandages, soaked in blood and pus. Dr Gupta was snapping orders, wrestling with the equipment. She saw Jamie's tibias and put her hand to her mouth. They were a creamy, ivory colour, not pure white like the bones you see in museums. (Display bones have been boiled and cleaned.) She had grown used to seeing his burn wounds but she'd never see living bones. She swallowed hard, trying not to cry.

Dr Gupta, his back to her, leaned over the bed, the other two standing back, hands on hips, their faces set, mouths clamped. Dr Gupta looked up and said something to Dave. Dave turned and started checking and adjusting the fluid and blood bags. Leaning against the glass, Shirley sniffed the air a couple of times. The whiff became a stench. She covered her mouth and nose to keep out the smell – the smell of her son's burning flesh. She kept her eyes on the scene, her mind a blank. After five minutes, Dr Gupta stood up straight, arched his back and exhaled hard, his cheeks blowing right out.

He turned to the door and, his face bursting with relief, gave Shirley a thumbs-up and a big grin. He didn't need to explain in words that disaster had been averted by a whisker. But he came outside and did exactly that while trying to draw the drama out of it, reminding himself he was talking to the mother not to a colleague, making out to her it was no big deal, *nothing to worry about, Shirley, all in a day's work, he's fine now* ... He explained how the arteries at the knees had sprung open, about hypovolemic shock being a life-threatening emergency, how the heart can't pump properly if there is rapid and severe loss of blood, how that can starve the organs of oxygen, damage the brain and the kidneys beyond repair ... but she was only half-listening because she was in a state of some sort of shock herself. She picked up just from the speed he was talking, the adrenaline still coursing through him, the intensity of their faces a few moments earlier, that the doctor was mighty relieved the procedure had worked and proud of his actions, that he could go home that evening happy in the knowledge he had saved a man's life.

9

Jamie's siblings, Ryan and Kimberley, came out during the second week. Shirley had been giving them regular updates on the mobile, sparing no detail on the extent of their elder brother's injuries. They knew what to expect – but the imagination wants to run only so far. It was a shock to see him in the flesh – or what they could see of him – that is, just the face, a face they may not have picked out in a line-up.

The living arrangements in the small room at Hubbard House became a little cramped and awkward, Shirley and Kimberley sharing the bed, Ryan camping among the suitcases. The good news was that not much happened during their visit. There was no drama. Jamie just lay in his bed, still as a felled tree, hanging in there. Occasionally, the medics took him down to theatre for a skin graft or to debride a limb and scrub off some mould. But there were no emergency episodes. He wasn't rushed into theatre, no one had to restart his heart with a defibrillator, no one was running or shouting, no alarm bells or sirens sounded. The machines bleeped and whirred, the tubes ran with fluids, the nurses and doctors came and went. It was nothing like an episode of *ER* or *Casualty*.

It was probably just as well that this appearance of stability was an illusion. For there was a great deal of drama taking place, all of it enacted in silence beneath the bandages. The bacteria were colonising, billions of microbes marshalling their forces, probing for a breach in the defences to storm through and run amok, looting and pillaging all the valuables until the besieged body lay in ruins. There were battles and skirmishes raging all over Jamie's body but warding off infection was the main front-line now, his own heavily compromised immune system doing what it could to shore up the resistance. The fungi kept growing back, the bacteria were forming up. Bacteria don't attack until they have sufficient forces so it was a question of picking them off and trying to keep them out of range. The pus drenching his bandages was the carnage left behind from the relentless attri-tional fight to keep the invaders at bay.

His body needed all the strength it could muster but it was dumping minerals and nutrients faster than the medics could replace them. Malnourishment is an inevitability and a major problem in severe burn trauma. The management of his fluids and electrolytes was closely and constantly monitored. The naso-gastric tube running down his oesophagus through his stomach into his duodenum was pumping a high-calorie, high-protein liquid feed into his system in vast quantities. The problem was that most of it was coming straight out and into the wound dressings. The extent of the burns had triggered a state of hypermetabolism – a stress response causing a huge acceleration of the chemical processes by which cells produce the substances and energy to sustain life.

That was normal for a body in Jamie's condition, but it was no less a danger for the knowledge of that. The treatment of malnutrition in patients suffering extreme body trauma is a poorly understood area of science even for experts in the field. Regimes vary widely from hospital to hospital and many ques-tions over the best form of nutritional delivery, the volume and composition of diet, were still to be answered satisfactorily.

So, for the better part of a week, Ryan and Kimberley came and went to Room Ten, oblivious to the drama playing out inside their brother. They were heartened that Jamie was still there every morning, silent and inert but ready to fight another day. He had survived the appalling inferno and crash and, like all acute conditions, the worst, it was logical to assume, was probably over. Shirley was relieved they had not been obliged to witness his descent into a critical emergency, as she had with the blood-loss episode. Or, heaven forbid, his death.

There was one shocking moment during their stay.

Shirley had taken over from the nurses the twice-daily task of cleansing Jamie's teeth and mouth. It was important that no germs built up in the oral cavity. The last thing he needed was pneumonia, the primary risk of a dirty mouth in an artificially vented coma patient. She'd press the button to raise the head of the bed, dip the swab in the antibacterial rinse and give his mouth a good going over.

One day she said to Ryan, 'How about you do his teeth this morning?' It was virtually impossible to help Jamie in a significant way, and Shirley understood that any such gesture of love or support allowed his brother and sister to feel as if they were making some sort of contribution to his recovery, however small. Everyone was helpless but desperate to help in whatever way they could. Many of Jamie's friends back in the UK did their bit by sending him play-lists of soothing, uplifting and nostalgic songs. Renee brought in her CD player and speaker from home for him and, overlaying the humming, whirring and bleeping of the life support machinery, the quiet music from Jamie's past washed around the room.

Happy to be of practical assistance after days of hanging around, Ryan took the swab and leaned over to open his brother's mouth. Jamie's eyes sprung open and, groggily, he asked, 'Mum, why aren't you doing it?' Then he shut his eyes and disappeared back into oblivion.

Ryan and Shirley were startled, standing there and looking at each other with wide eyes. It was like something out of a horror movie. They summoned Renee. She explained that what they had witnessed was not common but nor was it abnormal for a patient in an induced coma. It was no different to someone sleep talking, she said. The level of his consciousness was determined by the quantity of sedatives in his system. His care team could control his consciousness just as they could control the volume button on the CD machine – you just turn it up or down.

When his condition improved – Shirley liked Renee's use of 'when' over 'if' – they would even be able to bring him around for half an hour or so, then turn up the barbiturate volume and deliver him back to noddy-land before the pain kicked in. Like a drunk, he would be unaware of what he was doing or saying, and would probably talk nonsense, but to everyone else in the room the resurfacing into consciousness is a magical moment. For Shirley and Ryan right then, their own fright quickly gave way to a sense of elation and hope after the event. Jamie was still in there. He had spoken to them. He was aware of them.

Whether the presence of friends and family at the bedside is a hormonal-boosting comfort that makes any real difference to a coma patient's recovery is another question that science can't quite answer. Consciousness is a mysterious phenomenon. Tests on coma patients have produced interesting results. By imaging the brain and watching the neural responses to questions and conversations, scientists found that most people in a deep 'vegetative' state are unaware of their environment. But, and this took them aback, as many as 20 per cent of patients might hear and understand everything going around them. But for how long that awareness lasts in the mind is another matter. Quite what goes on in the grey matter of the comatose mind remains exactly that – a grey area.

Though very heavily sedated, Jamie had spoken a whole sentence, he had asked a sensible question, revealing his comprehension that it was his mother who usually brushed his teeth.

The episode got Shirley thinking. It begged the questions: So, what else was Jamie taking in? How much did he know? Were his emotions engaged? Was he being lifted by the love and support he was getting? By Shirley and Renee's upbeat, soothing chatter? Maybe he was one of the lucky ones – or maybe it was unlucky. Was it good for Jamie to hear all those gloomy prognoses pronounced, the sighing, the gasps and the sobbing?

When Ryan and Kimberley climbed into the cab and headed back to Orlando International, Shirley, standing outside Hubbard House, was experiencing mixed emotions. It had been great to have the three of them at his bedside, united in love and worry, and she was encouraged that Jamie might have been aware of their presence. But there was an element of relief that she could now go back to tending to Jamie, give him her full attention. No matter how much she might love them too, other people – offspring included – were a distraction from the only true focus of her attention: her child in the bed fighting for his life. Loving them all equally as she did, delighted they'd come out, she was happy to return to her routine: a clear room and a clear head meant clear focus and judgement.

• • •

As it soon turned out, Shirley needed all her wits about her and her faculties undisturbed by other thought. Then again, given what was developing, maybe she could have well done with the distraction and the comfort of her family about her.

An expert now in body language and facial expressions, the next morning Shirley knew as soon as she squeaked towards the nurses' station in her galoshes that something was up. Something really bad. Dave, the nurse on Jamie duty, was standing head down, eyes fixed on a screen. When he looked up and saw it was the mum coming his way, his lips puckered, his brow creased and he dropped his head back down. The medic's lip-pucker, she had learned, was effectively a red flag. As much as 75 per cent of our communication is said to be non-verbal, and Shirley was becoming fluent in body language.

She looked through the glass door to her left. Dr Smith and two nurses were in with Jamie.

Shirley said, 'Oh no, what now?'

'I better get Doctor Smith to explain.'

'Tell me.'

Dave lifted the laptop on to the counter, pressed some keys and spun it around. There was an X-ray of a chest. Shirley put her on her glasses. Ribs, spine, the broken collarbone and a mass of grey and white blotches came into sharp focus.

'Pulmonary effusions,' he said.

'What are they?'

'Pleurisy. Build-up of fluid between the lungs and the ribcage. The white patches on the lungs are the fluid.'

Shirley leaned into the screen. One of the lungs was virtually covered in white, the other half so.

'So what are the doctors going to do?'

'They're on it. They've draining the fluid away with tubes inserted into his chest.'

Shirley said, 'Oh good! So he's okay now then?'

'Er, not quite, Shirley. Here comes Doctor Smith. He's the expert.'

The smile that usually wreathed the diminutive doctor's face was not there that morning. There was not even a suspicion of one.

'What's going on, Doctor Smith?' She felt the alarm spread over her like a flesh-eating rash and her heart went cold.

His face was rumpled, the manner humble, the voice quiet as he spoke.

'Jamie has pneumonia.'

'Pneumonia! No!'

'Here, let's go somewhere quiet and I'll explain while the team sort out the antibiotics and fluids.'

He led her into a quiet room, holding the door and throwing out an arm in the direction of a chair.

It was almost inevitable Jamie would get pneumonia apparently, but, he explained, they had had no intention of burdening her with that grim possibility while she had so much else to worry about.

The risk of pneumonia, caused by bacteria in the system, is very high in severe burn patients with heavily compromised immune systems, he said. It often got into the blood stream during hospital procedures – catheters, intravenous equipment, gastric tubes, the intubation pipe in his throat. Jamie had all of those. It's called HAI pneumonia – a hospital acquired infection.

Jamie also had third-degree burns to 65 per cent of his body surface and, as she would no doubt recall from the amputation crisis, his exposed, damaged tissue offered a fertile breeding ground for bacteria. So, the bacteria that had triggered the pneumonia might have found its way in by any number of those routes.

Shirley was half-listening now. It didn't matter now. The fact was he had pneumonia. It was another emergency. You can die of pneumonia even if you're otherwise healthy. The risk of death increases significantly in the very elderly or the very unwell. Dr Smith did not need to add that Jamie was very unwell. She knew all that.

Shirley clasped her hands between her knees, staring the floor shaking her head. When was her boy going to catch a break? The assault on him was relentless and savage.

Dr Smith wasn't done.

'But the tough news, Shirley, I'm afraid, is ...'

'There's more?'

'The tough news is that Jamie has sepsis too.' He spat out the words, like he had to get it out there quickly, get it over and done with.

Shirley threw herself back in her chair, groaning at the ceiling. 'Dear God! Sepsis – that could kill him too, yeah? Isn't that right?'

'They are both life-threatening conditions, yes.'

'So, pneumonia, sepsis, sixty-five per cent burns, abdominal compartment syndrome, malnutrition, broken immune system, pleurisy, damaged colon and liver – how much more can he take? Why not throw in some Ebola? If this was a theory test in your medical exams, you'd answer that the patient was more likely to die than not. Correct?'

She was ranting a little but she couldn't help it. Her fight response was in full flow. Dr Smith gave her the sympathetic mouth-pucker and waggled an outstretched hand, making it seem like a 50–50 scenario but she could tell by his face Jamie's odds were way shorter.

'Maybe, maybe not, Shirley. Jamie has already shown quite extraordinary resilience. He is made of strong stuff – obviously comes from very good stock!'

Shirley appreciated the doctor's attempt at humour and kindness but the muscles in her face refused to give him a smile back.

'You're right, Doctor Smith! He's not going to die. I'm telling you that as a statement of fact. I know.'

'If he's got half your spirit, Shirley, he's sure got a good chance.'

'So, what are you doing, Doctor Smith?'

'Fluids and antibiotics – very aggressive antibiotic treatment.'

'How aggressive?'

'We had to throw everything at the problem, fast. Very fast. He was going into a septic shock – blood pressure dropping to lethal levels … high probability of multi-organ failure because the organs aren't getting any blood … leading to respiratory failure, cardiac arrest … Death is a matter of when, not if. You have to act on the spot. It's not a moment to go away and have a think about it, or even wait for you to get here. We are giving him the two strongest in very high doses.'

'What are the risks of such aggressive antibiotic use?'

'Relative to death?' Dr Smith shrugged and let the question answer itself.

• • •

Shirley went through to see Jamie. He looked much the same as he had done the day before except – and she may have been imagining it – his chest was rising and falling at a much faster rate. So was hers. She gently laid a latex glove on his good shoulder – or the better one at least – and spoke to him, urging him to be strong, that this was the absolute worst of it, that the antibios were going to knock it for six, that she was proud of his strength, that she loved him dearly …

When the physios came in to bend his joints, she made her way out into the mezzanine. Santa Claus gave her his lovely gentle smile. She smiled back, the best she could manage, and wondered if a snow-white beard and a comforting face were the only criteria for a job of sitting on reception in a trauma unit. Santa himself couldn't have done a better job of radiating warmth.

She took out her mobile and did what she had promised herself she would not do: she googled. She thumbed 'Pneumonia AND Sepsis Prognosis' into the search window. She trawled through the sites, page after page. None of them said, *He'll be right as rain in no time!* She slid the phone into her pocket and, taking the stairs, face and mind blank as a sleepwalker, made her way down to the chapel. Except when she was trying to sleep in Hubbard House, or in Room Ten at Jamie's side, the chapel was where she stayed: knees on the pew kneeler, chin on her clasped fingers.

10

Ever since Jamie's arrival on the helipad and the frantic battle to keep him alive in the days that followed, the Orlando team had been keeping an eagle eye on his kidneys.

Acute renal failure (ARF) is a common complication of severe burns and about 25 per cent of patients will die from it. Small advances have been made in understanding kidney problems in burns patients but there has been very little improvement in the mortality rate. The problems can arise at the very outset during the immediate resuscitation of the body fluids when the burns are fresh and the body is reacting ferociously to the all-out assault upon it. The fluid enables blood flow to the kidneys, but in a body badly charred or scalded, much of it leaks straight out of the damaged blood vessels and tissues. That means blood flow becomes poor. If 20 per cent of the body surface is severely burned, the blood flow to the kidneys will fall away, causing potentially lethal damage. The greater the burn area, the greater the insult to the kidneys. So, if 65 per cent is severely burned …

The Orlando reception team had pumped Jamie with fluids on his arrival in the trauma bay using a long-established measure known as the Parkland formula. It is difficult to get the balance right. Too little fluid early on will starve the kidneys of oxygen. But too much can be harmful as well, resulting in catastrophic respiratory problems, rapid bleeding and swelling of localised areas (life-threatening compartment syndromes) and pneumonia. In short, too much fluid can kill you. As it happened, Jamie was to suffer all those problems down the line but on that first day, he had reacted abnormally to his fluid resuscitation. His blood pressure plunged and he was pissing the fluids as fast as he was taking them on. The trauma team eventually stabilised the situation, his kidneys were saved, he was saved, and onwards his body and the medical team marched to the next battle.

The little bean-shaped organs tucked away halfway up the back, one either side of the spine, serve as a vital indicator of the body's status and performance – but they are vital in themselves too. In just a couple of minutes, the kidneys filter about two of the ten pints of blood circulating through your organs and around your body.

The kidneys may be small, about the size of a small fist, but they are tireless in the effort they put in for the body. If the heart and liver are the shire horses of our daily operation, doing the heavy pulling, with the brain the driver up top, our kidneys are our pack mules, carrying the essentials without which the rest cannot proceed with the journey. Our kidneys maintain the vital fluid balances of the body, regulating and filtering minerals from the blood, sifting out the waste materials from food, medications and toxins, expelling it as urine. They also create the hormones that help produce our red blood cells, promoting bone health and regulating blood pressure.

Your kidneys are your waste disposal system. Making sure the urine keeps flowing is not a glamorous job – no one pays the janitor too much attention. Until, of course, something goes wrong in the restrooms, like a blockage or there's a note on the door saying *Closed for Repairs until Further Notice*. The fact you can lose one and still live just as well and as long as a person with two has created the impression that kidneys can't be that important. How can they be if you can chuck one away and not notice the difference? It's true you can live a perfectly normal life with one kidney but you cannot lead a life at all with none. If the kidneys pack up, you pack up.

That's what Jamie's suddenly threatened to do while his body was hard at work battling pneumonia and sepsis on top of the primary injury and cause of all other problems – the burns themselves. Just when it seemed his devastated body could take no more punishment, his kidneys gave up the ghost, triggering yet another emergency in Room Ten. It wasn't the kidneys fault per se. They just weren't getting enough blood to work with.

Shirley was on her knees, literally and figuratively, when she got the call. Or rather, she got the vibrating buzz in her pocket while she was on the pew kneeler – and she raced from the chapel up to the third floor.

Jamie's team had been on high alert for this moment and, sure as night follows day, and sepsis follows pneumonia follows bacteraemia follows severe burns ... renal failure added its name to the burgeoning list of diagnoses on Jamie's records. Kidney injury is seen early on many in severe burns patients but it often occurs later on after sepsis has taken hold, triggering low blood pressure and generating an abundance of tiny blood clots. The blood flow to the kidneys is cut off and, without blood, their purpose in life is taken away from them, and they stop functioning. The worse the sepsis, the worse the kidney problem.

Jamie's urine flow had slowed to a trickle despite a steady stream of fluids. That was the first sign. Blood tests followed, but the doctors had guessed the results. They were going to show a rise in levels of serum creatinine – the waste product usually expelled by the kidneys. The normal range for creatinine in the blood is about 1 milligram per decilitre (one tenth of a litre). Anything over 1.3 is high. A reading of 5.4 is extremely high, indicating that significant kidney damage had already occurred. Jamie's was 5.4.

When kidneys fail, and the body loses its ability to clean out the blood and regulate its vital fluids and electrolytes, no other organ takes over the role. So, a dialysis system was wheeled at pace down the corridor to join the bank of life-support machinery in Room Ten. A dialysis machine is just an artificial kidney, connected to the body by tubing through a catheter. In Jamie's case, femoral catheters were inserted in his thighs, the route least favoured by surgeons because it's more prone to infection. But there was nowhere else on the body they could gain access to a major vein. He had tubes and wires hanging out every part of his body that hadn't been charred to the bone. Over the following weeks, 300 times a day, Jamie's blood, all 12 pints of it, would make the journey out of his body along the tubes and into the dialysis machine at the foot of his bed and back into his circulation, filtered and cleaned.

There was barely any part of his body, or its functions, that he could still call his own. The blood flowing through him belonged to a machine and the air he breathed to another machine; his food and liquids came from tubing feeds, his urine and stool went straight into bags, the skin grafted all over his body belonged to the deceased. And his brain, or his consciousness at least, had been put to sleep. He had ceased to be a human being. He had become the adjunct of machinery, a living receptacle for tubes, wires and powerful pharmaceuticals.

11

Two months after the accident, there he lay still in Room Ten, Burns Unit, Trauma Center, Orlando Regional Medical Center, a tangle of wires and tubes linking him to a crescent of sophisticated contraptions, a cross between Frankenstein's monster and the Six Million Dollar Man (for that was the approximate total cost of the trauma treatment to which he was heading).

The good news was that he was still refusing to die. He remained hypercritical but stable hypercritical. His face beneath the jellied veil was still a shocking sight for a mother to behold, the familiarity failing to stale the horror. Elsewhere on his ravaged body, black fungi and invisible bacteria continued to swarm and his system battled against waves of sepsis. The chest cavity kept filling with fluid, the tubes draining it away. The weeks went by and so he continued to breathe through the tube in his throat; the tubes of the dialysis machine hooked up to his thighs continued to run with his blood and fluids. Round and round it went, dirty blood out of the body, clean back in.

The plastic surgeons grafted and debrided as often as they felt his body could take the insult. But there was only so much of his good skin there to work with, only so much donor skin that matched his type, and owing to the stubborn mould in addition to the severe degradation of his regular bodily functions, the new skin struggled to take. They worked on his 'auto-amputated ears' to tidy up the mess of cartilage and necrotic tissue. They worked on the multiple lacerations to the face: his shattered nose, cheekbone, eye socket and mouth. The severe damage to the facial skin made the surgery for this highly complex.

Visitors came and went too, anxious on entering, even more so on leaving. Two old army mates, Pete Mash and Mark Brown, Terri, his on-off Canadian girlfriend, his father and siblings again, an aunt ... but he was none the wiser of their presence even when the nurses elevated the head of the bed to sit him up, eased off the sedative a little. Sometimes, looking at them blankly with his giant sunken fisheyes, no eyelids to blink behind the translucent mask, he began talking. It was just nonsense that spilled from his mouth and it was an unsettling experience for those in the room. Jamie was there but he wasn't, he appeared conscious but he wasn't. It was like talking to a man high on hallucinogens, the guy thinking he was making perfect sense, everyone else not sure how to respond. One day, Renee turned on the television and he watched an entire American football game, staring glassily at the screen like a lobotomy patient. He was never going to remember it. It was as much about the appearance of normality for Shirley's sake as real evidence of his progress.

It was all weird, it was worrying, it was wearying. How long was he going to stay like that? Even if he did come out of the coma for good, what then? What would he be like? What would he make of it all? Of his new self? How was this man of action going to rebuild his life as a man of inaction? A man who had rebuilt his life so impressively once already? What if he woke up properly and he was furious – furious they had kept him alive for a life that would no longer have meaning or purpose for him? Shirley tried not to think about it. She was doing what every mother would do, protecting and nurturing her offspring. It was better just to focus on the here and now than worry herself sicker about what the future might hold. The fact was that even two months on, death was still never more than a day or two away.

It was mid-October when she took the call in the middle of the night. She reached for the phone fearing the worst. It was the nurse on nightshift, the lovely Asian one. He was so happy, he was almost singing it down the line. 'Jamie's wet the bed! Jamie's wet the bed! His kidneys are working, Shirley!'

This was a major breakthrough because it showed that his body was regenerating, reclaiming tasks from the machinery.

The nurse told Shirley that they did a little dance by the central station. She put the phone down, leaped from bed and, pulling on her clothes, launched into her own song and dance.

'Jamie's wet the bed! Jamie's the wet bed!' she sang. After a minute, there was a knock on the door. It was the night porter.

'Is everything all right, Miss Kristensen?'

'Is everything all right? Is everything all right? You bet everything's all right, my friend. My son's just wet the bed! He's done the golden piddle.'

'That's wonderful news, ma'am. Good night.'

Part 3

Part I

12

9 November 2007

'Fuck off!'

Those were my first coherent words for three months – the first I remember uttering at any rate. It's the dimmest of memories.

The woman had a strong cockney accent and she was being firm with me. Sleep was pulling me back and I was aware of disappointing her somehow. There was a stench of kerosene. The wind was bitter. It's not hurricane season. Why's it so goddam cold? And what's with the kerosene? And that deafening noise?

'Come on, Jamie love, we've got to get you out of here and into the ambulance.'

'I want my American nurse.'

'You're not in America, Jamie love. You're in Essex. Stansted Airport. You're going to Chelmsford, my dear.'

Essex? What the … ? I drifted away, back into the dark depths.

I wish I could report that I had dropped into the world of the living for a moment and exclaimed, *Woohoo, I'm alive! … Peace, joy and love to you all!*

But no. I said, *Fuck off*. Nice, thanks for popping in, Jamie.

That was in November. I was given a second chance to try out my coma manners about five or six weeks later. This time I was awake for a while longer – the first prolonged period since the accident, a few minutes in all, and I was vaguely aware of what was going on around me, my brain fighting hard in a cloud of confusion to work it all out. It was getting on for Christmas and it was the day I was considered stable enough to be taken from the Intensive Care Unit (ICU) to the stepdown ward – an intermediate level for patients on the rung between there being a strong risk of dying and a strong risk of surviving.

They had been reducing the sedative levels over a few days and slowly the world had been coming into very dim focus. It was still a great pea-souper of a fog that blanketed my small world, but occasionally a shaft of light would break through and I'd get a snapshot of my surroundings – a nurse's face maybe, the bleeping of a machine, a snatch of conversation, each of these tiny moments of consciousness accompanied by a sensation of enormous pain being held back by the dull fuzz of medication. Anyhow, I guess that was the day I should have heard the church bells pealing in my head, a dawn chorus of birdsong filling my soul. I was alive! I'd done it! I had survived that terrible inferno! I'm getting my life back!

But once again I registered a very low reading on the joys-of-spring counter.

'Wakey, wakey, Jamie!' sung the nurse. 'Wakey, wakey! Rise and shine!'

'Piss off!'

'Now, now, Jamie, there's a good lad. We're taking you to the stepdown ward. It's a big day. A happy day.'

'Piss off!'

I remember desperately wanting to go back to sleep.

'Come on, Jamie love, we've got to get you going.'

'Who are you? You're not my American nurse! I want my American nurse.'

The painkilling meds must have been dropped pretty low because I was in a great deal of pain all over. Pain, I was going to find out, is the price I had to pay for consciousness. If I wanted the pain to go away, I had to get them to pump up the meds and I'd head back to la-la land. They were trying to advance my recovery, get me out of the coma, start doing things for myself. It was all part of the rehab programme. Fair enough. But no one volunteers for pain. Worse still, being conscious also meant being aware of my condition, thinking about my future. Right then, I just wanted to go back to sleep. Sleep's great. You don't have to think or feel.

'No, Jamie, there are no American nurses here. We're all Essex girls.'

She said it with a laugh in that nice cheery, cheeky way nurses can have about them.

So, they got me to the stepdown ward and I was wheeled into my room with all these machines attached to me. It was very cold, at least it felt very cold to me. There were a few Christmas decorations here and there in the corridors, some tinsel around a noticeboard, a stumpy plastic tree with some crappy paper rings. My mind was trying to compute: Yesterday, Florida and incredible summer heat, today Essex and incredible cold. Hmm. Then a flash of memory – the kerosene, Stansted. Oh yeah, I am back in England. I had a plane crash and caught fire.

Later that day, when I came round again, Mum was sitting at my bedside. I had been conscious of her lately, but I hadn't *seen* her since midsummer. I said, 'I defied the devil, Mum!' Or rather, I groaned it, my head flopped over, mouth dribbling.

She said, 'Yes you did, my boy, yes you did.'

I had half an eye open and she was standing now, her hand on my bandages and there were tear streaks on her cheeks.

Every now and then a shaft of light cut through the darkness, the truth slowly coming into focus. Yes, I was in Essex. The St Andrews Centre for Plastic Surgery and Burns, to be precise, part of the Broomfield Hospital in Chelmsford. I was no longer in Florida. It was no longer summer. It was Christmas. My reawakening was gradual and piecemeal, just the odd snatch of an insight before I'd sink back down again into the darkness. Sliding back, I saw myself as a drowned body bobbing to the surface from time to time.

Over the weeks, the windows of awareness grew longer and wider, my mind clearing ever so slowly, like a heavy sea fog being burned off by a weak sun, just failing to break through. I began the long process of piecing together what had happened to me, the state I was in. I have never much liked jigsaws and this mental version of one, picturing my state of being, contained a thousand tiny pieces.

Almost every time I 'woke up', Mum was at my bedside and the longer I was able to keep from falling back to sleep, the more she was able to explain what had happened. She didn't tell me everything at first. She was clever like that. She didn't want to hit me with it all in one hideous blast of information. She just fed morsels about my condition, about the treatment and all the operations. I picked up insights from the nurses and doctors too but it wasn't until the New Year that I had gained a strong understanding on what had been going on for almost five months.

Five months of my life gone, completely erased from my life! Had I really been lying motionless in a bed all that time? Dozens of strangers cutting, scraping and stitching my body, swabbing, washing, anointing and dressing me, exercising me, piercing me with tubes, wiring me with cables, swathing me in bandages over and over, emptying my waste, taking me for rides down corridors and lifts, probing and examining, standing around me rubbing their chins and discussing my chances? And not just medics but family and friends too, dozens of them, sitting at my bedside, sighing and chatting to me, some of them sobbing? Mum says that in Orlando I even watched a whole game of American football. Weird.

Weird because it seemed like yesterday that I was rolling around in the grass on fire. In a way, it was I suppose. I remembered the flames raging around me in the cockpit as though it had only just happened. I remembered my anger at the dumb mechanic or whoever it was had screwed up my engine and wrecked my life. I remembered standing on the wing of the plane, the fire like a flamethrower down one side of me, the massive thump on hitting earth, the deafening noise and the immense blast wave of the explosion. I remembered the two guys screaming at me to hang in there. The pain! Jesus. I remembered the whop-whop-whop and the downdraft of the chopper blades. I remembered shouting at the doctors in their scrubs on the hospital roof to kill me. And I remembered that image – stuck in my mind the whole time before someone stuck the needle in and gave me the sweet stuff. The image so strong it was almost a reality: me as a burning little mouse hanging by the thinnest of threads connected to heaven.

No kidding – it was like it had all taken place just a few hours previous, like I had just had my big bowl of muesli and was bouncing along in the Florida sunshine, through the golf course, happy as a skylark, looking forward to becoming a fully qualified pilot and in a couple of days heading back to the UK and then off for the greatest of my life challenges, fighting in a war. But no, five months had passed and I was bedbound in Essex, bandaged like an Egyptian mummy, wired up like Frankenstein's monster. That really wasn't how the day was meant to pan out. By rights, in terms of conscious hours passed since getting airborne, I should now be sitting around a barbeque with a beer in my hand watching the big Florida sun sink over the horizon.

And what had been happening in the wider world? How had the lads and the regiment been getting on? Had new wars broken out? Was Gordon Brown still Prime Minister, George W. Bush still President? Were my grandparents still alive?

The doctors in Florida had been in no hurry to be rid of me, Mum said, but the insurance company back in the UK couldn't get me out of there fast enough. Fair dos – the bills were enormous apparently, running to millions, because the care I was receiving there was out of this world. She said the phone calls from the man from the insurance company in the UK became more frequent and more desperate. The guy had the underwriters on his back, he kept telling her, and they were doing their nut about the soaring costs. Poor guy! Pretty well as soon as I was stabilised – critical still but stabilised – at immense expense, the insurance people booked a special aircraft and flew me out of US airspace. If they'd had the rocket ship to do it, they would have flown me over the Atlantic at the speed of light. The moment they got me into the free treatment of the NHS could not come soon enough.

Mum didn't tell me I had been as good as dead for the first two months, that I had touched the other side endless times. I worked that out, reading between her lines. Nor did she tell me I was still a long way from being out of the woods, but I didn't need a PhD in pathology to work that out either. Apart from a brain haemorrhage, a burst aorta or the Ebola virus, it seemed that, laid up over there in Orlando, I had just about every other life-threatening condition left on the list. Anywhere else but that amazing burns unit, I would have been a goner, she said. It was unbelievable what they did for me. As soon as it was physically possible, I was determined to go back there and thank them in person. But that day, if it was ever to come, was a long way off. That was blindingly obvious. I wasn't going anywhere in a hurry. Just getting out of bed and walking to the toilet was a long way down my things-to do-next-year list.

In Florida, someone called Dr Howard Smith had been my saviour, my lead consultant, she said – I think Mum had developed a bit of a soft spot for him, the way she spoke about him – but my guardian angel was a gorgeous strawberry blonde with a cute fringe called Renee. She loved me apparently, looked after me like I was her own child. Mum reckoned we'd make a great couple. Tough, no bullshit, but full of love and goodness. So, it was *her* voice going around and around my head. Still going around. I have no solid memories of my time in Orlando Regional Medical Center, just that lovely haunting voice. I don't remember any of the words riding on that voice, but the sound of it was like a warm rug, a tight embrace. You wonder what she saw in me lying there all messed up, like half-fried mince.

Why was her voice my only memory, or rather my only sensation of memory? Or should that be a memory of a sensation? It's hard to describe an experience that wasn't really an experience at all. You know those dreams – you wake up knowing you've had a powerful one, so strong it feels like something happened to you for real. But you can't remember a single detail. It's just a big, powerful feeling. That's how it felt with this voice. If I closed my eyes and she was there physically at my side again I'd recognise the voice straight off. I can't say that this Renee saved my life, but what I can say is that her gorgeous voice somehow kept me connected with the world, all that time in my darkness. Maybe I was fighting for her. Maybe I fancied her and wanted to impress her by surviving. Who knows? And maybe the reason I don't remember Mum's voice was because it is so familiar to me. You expect your Mum to be there. But you don't expect to hear the voice of a strange woman. The voice of that strange woman was like a hand reaching out across the void hanging on to mine for dear life.

● ● ●

It's interesting to find out what you've been up to for five months. Check this out – on 9 November 2007, my last day in Orlando,

I'm still in my coma, of course, and they put me in a great big padded chair and, still hooked up to a bunch of machines, I'm wheeled out to the nurses' station. All the doctors and nurses are there, crowding around me. Mum says they were all smiling and clapping, and that Renee was welling up. They were so proud. You've got to love Americans. I can't think of a nation that loves and sanctifies life more, so uncynical and shameless in their joy of being alive. These medics just couldn't believe I'd made it – or made it that far at least. It was down to them that, almost three months on, I was there in that big chair, not in the cold earth of a windswept graveyard back in Hertfordshire.

Mum was smiling and clapping back at them, overwhelmed with gratitude. She said my medical records would fill a room. They had done so much for me, 24 hours a day for three months, up and down the lift, in and out of the operating theatre, about a dozen specialists from different departments, all of them all over my case. Over and over they pulled me back from the brink and in between they kept patching me up – literally – as best they could.

I was flown home in a Learjet formerly owned by the King of Denmark but it was probably just as well I had no idea I was back in an aircraft, royal or otherwise, my last flight having not turned out so well. The ambulance raced out of downtown Orlando, sirens wailing, lights spinning, and we were waved straight through the gates in the far corner of Orlando International.

The repatriation company laid on their own nurse and, strapped tight into a narrow portable bed with all my machines around me, I was wheeled out to the aircraft from the hangar area, raised on a special lift and slotted through the loading hatch. There were two pilots and one air stewardess, and her only job was to look after Mum in her leather cream seat that a queen used to sit in. My mum deserved nothing less. She had been there for me day in, day out. (At least, unlike her, I was oblivious to the nightmare of those months. She lived it.) My bed and all my equipment were secured down one side.

There was no hanging around. Within minutes, the little luxury jet was screeching down the runway and we were away, straight into the same airspace from where I had enjoyed my last view of the world before it all went pear-shaped: the never-ending beach, the glistening surface of the ocean and those puff-balls of cloud in the bright blue sky. *Goodbye Florida, it's been nice.*

Mum says we stopped in Goose Bay, Canada, to refuel: the aircraft with kerosene, her with a Magnum ice cream given to her by the handsome pilot. So, I've been to Goose Bay now. Thirty minutes later, we were airborne again, heading up towards Greenland and the Arctic Circle. An ambulance was waiting for us on the runway at Stansted and – after telling the nurse to fuck off – I was hurried into it and blue-lighted at terrifying speed, according to Mum, to Broomfield Hospital.

You wouldn't have guessed it to look at me but I was considered to be stabilised by the time I was flown back. By that they meant only that I hadn't experienced some sort of life-threatening emergency for over a couple of weeks. I had taken the first steps into the foothills of the mountain I must scale to reach my recovery, its peak currently lost to view. I hadn't even reached base camp and it was but a short tumble back to the bottom, laden as I still was with the heavy baggage of all my conditions.

Six or seven weeks on, now in the stepdown ward, the sedatives were eased down, the pain rising in step with my increasing powers of awareness through the haze of meds. I was vaguely alert and I was asking Mum for more details about what had happened in Orlando, trying to add a few more pieces to the jigsaw on the blank surface of my memory. Mum dug out a copy of my discharge summary the Orlando team had written up for her future reference and for their colleagues in Chelmsford. The serious diagnoses, worthy of record, were: deep third-degree, 60–69 per cent body burn, severe sepsis, septicaemia, septic shock, traumatic abdominal compartment syndrome, acute respiratory failure, acute post-haemorrhagic anaemia, multiple pleural effusions, mycoses, acute renal failure, glucocorticoid deficiency, hyposmolality, bacterial pneumonia, protein and calorie malnutrition, acidosis, urinary tract infection, thrombocytopenia ... I'd never heard of most of them, had no idea what they meant, and there were other, lesser causes for concern, secondary matters related to the main events.

Strangely, the summary didn't list the ruptured liver and colon, I guess because they came under the heading of abdominal compartment syndrome. The broken bones weren't mentioned either. They had their own separate document, Mum said, moving on to list the theatre operations and procedures I underwent. After about three dozen, I asked her to stop. I got the picture. The upshot of all that clinical effort and surgical endeavour was that roughly half of the 65 per cent of my burn sites had been covered with new skin by the Orlando plastic surgeons. That, however, didn't include my donor sites from which they had harvested some of the good stuff.

So, five months on, in total just under half of my body surface remained unhealed, my immune system heavily compromised still. Consequently, bacterial and fungal infection persisted as a major threat to my existence. British hospitals were riddled with MRSA at the time and the battle against this invasive multi-resistant plague had been going on for years. Before I had gone to Florida, it was often front page in British newspapers, thousands of inpatients dying from infection, mostly the elderly and those, like me, in the very high-risk groups. There's never a good time to get MRSA, but late 2007, early 2008, was especially poor timing.

I was, at least, in good hands, or good latex surgical gloves. The Broomfield Burns Unit was one of the best in the country for severe cases and I had two of the best practitioners in Dr Peter Dziewulski and Dr Odhran Shelley overseeing my case. It was a happy coincidence that Dziewulski had trained under Dr Howard Smith from Orlando.

Shelley went to work on my face a few weeks after my arrival. He certainly had his work cut out. Much of it he performed in one major operation. Mum told me it made a huge difference to my appearance, especially around the eyes. Since the accident, my eyes appeared to be sitting at slightly different levels to each other. With no eyelids, the eyeballs looked huge and, owing to the shattered bone on one side and the burned flesh on both, they also gave the impression of having sunk into and slid down my cheeks. Hey kids, why are you running away?

I say 'Mum told me' because no one would hold up a mirror to me. I knew it wasn't going to be a pretty sight but I was morbidly fascinated to see how much the accident had changed me – curious in the same way that we slow down for a gawp at a road accident, or make ourselves sit through a really macabre horror movie. I was in no state to go and find a mirror for myself.

This wish to know what I looked like built into an urgency. You can cover the rest of your body with clothes but not your face. Even an armed bank robber takes off his balaclava when he gets home. The face is who you are. Clothes and hand gestures are secondary when it comes to immediate impressions. The face is our passport. It's what we present to the world. It's how people recognise us or, in my case, how they might not. The face is the principal instrument in our communication toolkit. Before we have opened our mouths to speak, the other person has looked at our face and formed their impression. They have worked out the mood we're in, the warmth or hostility, the surprise or disappointment, all expressed with a few almost imperceptible tugs of the facial muscles. You can say the sweetest words in the world but if it looks like you're snarling at me, I'm out of there or bracing for a scrap. If your faces light up at the sight of me, I'll be right in there shaking your hand or giving you a hug. What if my face could no longer perform these basic tasks of human interaction that we all take for granted? What if it was just a blank, rough canvas or, worse, a Halloween mask?

My teeth, along with my penis, were the only part of my body to be unaffected by the work of the flames and, later, by the work of the surgeons in the harvesting festival performed on what good skin had been left. My face had taken a fearful battering from flame and fall, and whatever magic the surgeons Dziewulski and Shelley and their team might work, how could I be sure my smile was ever going to come across kindly and not as a sneer, or a straight-up canine baring of the teeth? Like I was growling at you? When we smile, we smile with the eyes too. The whole face lights up. What if mine could no longer do that despite all the hard graft of the plastic surgeons? What if my face was just smeared putty with a hole for eating and breathing, two little ones for more breathing and two big fish eyes?

I used to be quite vain. I was a good-looking lad and I never had trouble getting along with beautiful girls. But so what now? Male grooming, the latest in clothes? Do me a favour. Coming around, romance and fashion were not preoccupations, even if my American nurse had managed to excite some feelings of love and longing from the other side. No, you quickly forget about love and other life luxuries when trying not to die is the main focus. Whenever I did bob into consciousness from the dark depths, my mind going for a wander, I was anxious as to how my appearance might affect others and how, in turn, that was going to bounce back on me and affect day-to-day living. That was the worry.

But appearance was the lesser anxiety. My main concern was my mobility, my new physical capabilities and limits as and when I was well enough to get up and start walking lessons. Walking lessons! That was what was truly freaking me out. I used to run ten miles for laughs, now I'd have to be coached to put one foot in front of the other.

I guess it was not surprising that my thoughts were mired in such pessimism, ever drifting towards despair, increasingly expressed in irritability and fretfulness. It was hard to find reasons to be cheerful. Surviving the accident, being alive to tell the tale, was not doing it for me. It was all dark in there. I did not see the palest glimmer of happiness or feel the lightest brush of hope. On the contrary. The happiness radar was blank and silent. It sat there like me, inert and useless. The last genuine moment of happiness I had experienced was in the cockpit of the plane looking out over the sparkling Atlantic below the perfect blue sky and thinking out how well my life was turning out. The awful thing was that it still felt like yesterday and that happiness had been a physical sensation.

The drugs made me feel down but they were a necessary evil to control the pain. Without them, I'd be screaming. I was clear-headed enough to understand that not all the dark thoughts running through my head deserved respect. I was lucid enough to know that they were the consequence of physical, chemical, hormonal influences on my mind. I got all that. I got too that, if I could just park the gloom and think rationally, think my way through the dull miserable haze – think clearly under pressure as they used to tell us in the army – then I could start on conjuring up a future for my new self. That would be a reward in itself, a positive activity, reversing the direction of the furious downward spiral of negative contemplation, turn that vortex into a virtuous tornado of hope.

I had turned my life around once already, and even though the nature of my condition first time around was more chronic than acute, it had been a long haul and a major effort. I had gone from street corner scumbag and petty criminal to university graduate, commissioned officer and instructor in almost any outdoor activity you care to name. So, let's do that again, I was saying to myself, surprise myself once more. Come on, let's build a third life and I promise to forget about becoming a pilot! Is that a deal?

But this time, thinking it through rationally, going through the possibilities, trying to make plans only made the outlook bleaker. There was no escaping the conclusions of a cold analysis of the prospects and possibilities. I could forget about the army, forget about skiing, forget about mountaineering, forget about scuba diving – my diving! I loved my diving – forget about outdoor adventure, forget about any endurance pursuit at which I used to excel. I could forget about all the activities I used to love. I could forget about the life I had.

So, assuming I regained a certain amount of mobility and physical capability, what to do? I hadn't been blessed with the brains of Stephen Hawking and I had never been able to sit still for a minute unless I was in an aircraft, a train or car knowing I was heading off for an adventure or a bout of manic activity somewhere. I had never felt comfortable in a chair.

In short, a question was starting to form in my mind: was mine a life worth saving, worth living? Was it really worth that immense clinical effort and cost, all that labour, all that fretting of family and good friends, if the end result was a guy whose meaningful life had effectively been taken away from him and left him with a body like a patchwork quilt, a mobility problem, and a face like a crème brûlée?

13

Lying there, there's little to do but think, to remember, go travelling in my mind. I'm going over my life all the time, like it's the end of it. Which, in a way, it is. I'm dreading my journey into the future, and the present sucks, staring at walls and ceilings, fuzzy on meds, my whole body tense and throbbing, never giving me a moment's respite. But the past is a happy place to visit, so I fly off there whenever I'm conscious, and sneak back there in my dreams too. I become a frequent traveller, my imagination racking up the air miles day after day, hour after hour.

I keep returning to the other truly momentous day in my life, just under seven years earlier in September 2000. It's Freshers' Fair at the University of East Anglia (UEA), a day that will throw my life in a completely different direction. Unlike 19 August 2007, this day is the making, not the breaking, of me, though I have no notion of that at the time. I am wandering through the stalls, checking out the multitude of societies and clubs to join. It's a proud moment – and an exciting one, marking as it did the start of a new life, an academic life, at a top university too. Had I told them I was an undergraduate studying Scandinavian languages, all my Leighton Buzzard mates, my teachers and the local cops would have laughed me into next week. But it was a fact, and even I had difficulty in accepting the truth of it. A few years earlier, I was trouble, hunting down a bad life.

Christ, I messed up my teenage years, way more than your average wayward adolescent. Or my teenage years messed up me.

Maybe it was a bit of both. Who knows? Who cares now? It's just fruitless navel-gazing. Whatever. I'd come through it. I survived.

It all began when my parents' rocky marriage finally collapsed. I was 12 when Mum left our home in Plantation Road, taking with her my baby sister Kimberley. That left just the three males – me, my dad Mick and brother Ryan, two years my junior. I loved my mum and I was distraught, and it didn't seem right that Dad should be abandoned. But I was still going to see my mum and speak to her all the time. So I stayed put. The problem was that Dad, a long-distance, heavy haulage driver for P&O Ferries, was out on the road for most of the week. In his absence, I, a 12-year-old, became head of the household. You could get away with that in the mid-1980s. That meant that I got myself and my brother ready for school, and off we went. Back in the afternoon, I prepped supper for the two of us then crashed in front of the telly or hit the streets to play with our mates. Dad always made sure there was food in the house and he gave me a little pocket money for doing the cleaning. Mum was on the phone all the time, checking in on her boys. It was working. The house didn't burn down, social services never knew – probably didn't care. We attended school, we went through the motions like the other kids, just without parents around. But ...

The new arrangements meant that I was growing up fast, maybe too fast. Gradually, boyish mischief turned to misdemeanours. Stealing sweets and little toys from corner shops became a regular habit. I started smoking, my cigarettes funded from the proceeds of more lucrative ill-gotten goods, sold around the school. After a year or so, cider and weed became a part of my lifestyle and there was to be the occasional venture into the harder stuff. You didn't need to be a child psychologist to work out that it wouldn't be long before the misdemeanours were upgraded to more serious offences and anti-social behaviour. In the space of a couple of years, I had graduated from standing around on street corners in an oafish gang to criminal damage and robbery. I was on my way up in the criminal world – and showing bags of promise.

I was short on conscience but not on confidence. If I wanted something, I just stole it. I quickly discovered I had quite a gift for theft. To be a good thief, you need balls, cunning and a healthy dose of indifference to the consequences. I had the lot, and in abundance. My folks had brought me up strictly, hammering me if I ever stepped out of line. I still shudder at the memory of the day Mum worked out I'd been pinching loose change from her purse. But my folks weren't there now. The fear of punishment had vanished, the testosterone levels of the adolescent were on the rise, and a who-gives-a-fuck attitude consumed my outlook on life.

Woolworths on the High Street was a sitting duck. Too quick and wily for the dozy security guard, I pretty well helped myself to whatever I fancied. Watches were good: they were small and relatively expensive. Woolies was just too goddam easy for an aspiring Artful Dodger – where was the thrill? – and the goods were so cheap that the returns were small. WHSmith was a cinch too but it wasn't much good for anything but sweets and stationery. Not many kids I knew were in the black market for Curly Wurlys and a pricey fountain pen.

So, bored of the lower leagues, I upped my game and the new focus of my criminal enterprise became Leighton Buzzard's main toyshop, on a little side street off the town centre. At first, I stole from it in broad daylight. Skateboards fetched good money and so did remote-control cars, and I had no fear of lifting them from under the nose of the hapless proprietor and his teenage shop assistants. Refining my reconnaissance and planning skills, I worked out that the toyshop was not overlooked by any other building and there was no alarm system. So, my mate and I started breaking in at night, shinning up the drainpipes, removing the tiles from the roof and breaking through the shop's panelled ceiling. I had climbed every tall tree in his neighbourhood, I was nimble, strong and I had no fear. It was a low ceiling and a short drop on to the shop floor. This shop was an Aladdin's cave and we'd carry off sacks of boxes, like evil little Santas, put the panel and the tiles back in place, bury the merchandise in woods down by the railway track, wait a week or two, then flog off the bounty. We even wore gloves and balaclavas. We considered ourselves pros – albeit pros with soprano voices and no pubes. We did that three times, decent intervals between each, before having the criminal sharpness to give the place a rest when the owner called in the cops and ramped up his surveillance.

So, we did a bank instead. I noticed that one of the High Street banks had a flat roof – an open invitation to a couple of fearless hoodlums so, easy as the toyshop, up we went up and made a hole. The only reason we didn't make the drop that night, so we told each other as we peered down into it, was because all the cash would be kept in a safe overnight. In truth, we knew we had gone too far. We were shitting ourselves. For a young lad, an unguarded toyshop was one thing, but one of Britain's leading banks was quite another. But we had got our thrills and given two fingers to the authorities and the world of dumb grown-ups, so I slipped home through the shadows to smoke a fag, watch some post-watershed telly, make sure my brother Ryan was tucked up safely in bed and do the cleaning before Dad got back from the road the next day.

I got caught only twice. Once, after robbing a calligraphy pen from WHSmith in Milton Keynes, I was literally collared by PC Plod – lifted off the ground by him like a shot rabbit. I was carted off to the lock-up until Dad arrived to deliver the mother of all rollickings. On the second occasion, my mate and I were caught in the act when, for a third day, we returned to the local garden centre to throw stones on to the roof of the glasshouse. God, that was fun, hearing all that glass shatter! This time, half-a-dozen employees were waiting for us, springing from the undergrowth as we unleashed our first hail of projectiles. I was cautioned for criminal damage.

The mounting delinquency took its toll on my performance at school. I was strong on arithmetic, probably from working out the potential proceeds from a robbery, but not much else. Sport was the one discipline at which I excelled. I loved it. I was a natural athlete and I had massive respect for the Sports teacher, Mr Cox. 'Coxy' treated me like an equal, or at least someone worthy of some respect. But my trips to smoke fags down in the woods by the narrow-gauge railway line became more frequent and the sport began to tail off.

In class, I was always exhausted from my nocturnal adventures and spent most of the time at the back, giving and receiving Chinese burns with my fellow ne'er-do-wells. In the playground, I wasn't shy of a fight and I was tidy with my fists. Only once did I come off the worse, picking a scrap with the toughest kid in the school, a wild animal of a child, and big too. It taught me a lesson: pick your fights wisely.

It was lucky that drugs didn't sit well with my troubled mind. I kept trying to join in the weed smoking with my mates but it just made me paranoid and sullen. When I succumbed to peer pressure and took acid, it was a horrifying experience. I dropped the tab under my tongue, but when nothing happened after an hour or so, I said goodbye to my mate, and went home to bed. Half an hour later I was curled up in a ball under the bedsheets, cowering from the fire-eyed goblin pressed against my bedroom window. *It was just a bad trip, mate, you were unlucky,* I was told. So I had another go. This time the walls I was climbing started to melt into toxic slime. So from then on, I stuck to the fags and booze.

Proof that I had completely wasted the years from 12 to 16 came in the late summer of 1991 when I tore open the brown envelope on the doormat and read that I had failed all but one of my GCSE examinations. A single 'C' was all I had to show for ten years of schooling. The rest were graded D to F. I stared at the slip of paper like I was watching a reel of film capturing in Technicolor my four years of waywardness and lost opportunities. I was thunderstruck, crushed by the scale of my failure. It was probably out of guilt for their absence in that period that my folks did not come down too hard on me. I was expecting to be bawled out, but I got nothing of the sort. Dad just put his arm around me and when I went to see Mum, she gave me a tearful hug. 'I'm sorry, my love. What are we going to do with you?'

What they did do was send me to Sixth Form College in nearby Dunstable where I had to drop a year and retake my GCSEs. This time I passed them all and, incredibly, I moved on to A levels. I still stood at a fork in the road because the college was split in two, with the good lads on one side of the divide and the bad lads on the other. And some of them were very bad, a few of them soon graduating to jail or heroin, or both. I had a foot in each camp but, gradually, witnessing my own improvement, I took up with the good guys, or the better ones at least.

At the weekends and in the holidays, I chose to work rather than rob. I quickly learned that hard work came with a double reward, paid out in pounds and in rising self-esteem. I started with paper rounds, graduated to supermarket work and finally on to quite a responsible post with a car security firm that manufactured locks and devices for road wheels and steering wheels. The boss, a bad-tempered Irishman, was a hard taskmaster but he was utterly fair if you put your back in. So that's what I did, and I was repaid with the man's respect and a wallet full of wedge. I was learning about graft and discipline.

My A-level grades were B, B, C – not magnificent, but 'good enough for government work' and way better than any of my former teachers would ever have predicted. I had given myself a fighting chance, some options, but first I wanted to get the hell out of bloody Leighton Buzzard.

And I went as far as I possibly could. I bought myself a British Airways round-the-world ticket and headed to Australia via a three-month working tour of southern Africa. It was in Australia that I discovered my passion – scuba diving – a passion that became almost an obsession and, over the years, was going to take me all over the world, to some of its most inaccessible regions, to the sites of some of the toughest dives. One day – thank God I didn't know at the time – this love of the world under the waves was going to have to save me from near-fatal despair.

I thought seriously about becoming a full-time diving instructor in Australia – all that sun and coral and all those girls and bars had generated a temptation almost beyond endurance. But I wasn't done achieving. I had the taste for it now. I was turning my life around and the wheel was still spinning. I returned to the UK and got a proper job.

My choice of career would have come as a serious surprise to my teachers and parents, and even more so to my new employers. I joined the police – Thames Valley Police – and ended up stationed in the very building in Milton Keynes in which I had been held for shoplifting as a tiny teenage tearaway. There was an element of looking for full redemption in my decision: to draw a very thick line under my wayward past. There was probably no longer a record of my misdemeanours in their files, but I confessed to them all the same, cleared my conscience, and hoped that the revelation showed I was playing it all by the book now. The recruitment people ummed and ahhed but, in my interview, the Chief Constable said he was impressed by my honesty and courage and they took me on.

I took to my role as a frontline patrolman with the same gusto I had taken to crime, haring around the town and the Buckinghamshire countryside, sirens wailing, blue-lights spinning, often on my own in the small hours when I was the only duty officer available.

It was exciting, adrenaline-pumping work and I threw himself into it day after day. But the cycle was repetitive, relentless and, ultimately, soul-crushing for a young man of growing ambition and self-confidence. Apprehending lowlifes was not the high life. I needed a break from breaking up pub fights, restraining violent drunks, visiting crash scenes, intervening in domestic abuse scenarios – and collaring teenage scallies for High Street shoplifting. And I missed my diving.

I knew I was held in high regard by my seniors but I had no high hopes that my request for a sabbatical would be granted. I had only been in post for three years. I was just chancing my arm, keeping my options open, so I was astonished when the Chief Super told me how much I was valued, that a rapid rise up the ranks awaited me ... on my return. He told me I could take up to three years!

So, for a second time, I toured the world, this time in a series of trips rather than one continuous adventure. I did nothing but dive, working my way up the Professional Association of Diving Instructors' ladder, earning money from my greatest passion and visiting exotic locations in the Near and Far East: Egypt on the Sinai and further down the Red Sea, Israel, Philippines, Micronesia.

There was now a proper career to be made in diving should I want it and I gave it serious thought. But that wheel of fortune was still spinning, my outlook widening, my confidence mushrooming. I had joined the police partly as form of penance, a way of erasing the sins of his past. Something similar but deeper was driving me on now. Yes, I had taken the right path in the end, turning away from the low-road signposted to hard drugs, heavy drinking, pub fights, high crime and jail. Those were destinations to which I would never take a detour now. Yes, I had taken the high road, the harder road, but still, the question remained ... what else could I make of myself? How much further could I push himself?

So, I flew home, took the train down to Norwich and enrolled at UEA. And as I wandered through the 200 stalls of the Freshers' Fair that day, all those societies confirmed my growing belief that the world was my oyster – I could do anything I wanted. I didn't have to stop at the first stall I came to, just as I didn't have to take the first career I chose and stay with it for the rest of my life. I could have joined the chess club, the salsa dancers, the philosophy society, the skateboarding society, the real ale drinkers, the athletics club, the canoeists, any number of charity, volunteer and campaigning groups. Damn it, I could have joined the feminist book club! Picking myself out of the gutter and getting myself educated had delivered the world to my doorstep. If I had enough focus and grit, I could make of this life whatever I wanted.

And I was soon to discover, as were my superiors, that will, strength of character and sheer bloody-minded determination were something I possessed in abundance. Because the only stall I stopped at was being manned by the Cambridge University OTC, the Officer Training Corps. The Cambridge branch welcomed UEA students, being in the same neighbourhood, and it had always been one of the most highly regarded in the country.

I had never given the Armed Forces a thought – Jamie Hull from Leighton Buzzard, an officer of the British Army? Do me a favour.

I picked up the literature and a fresh-faced lad in crisp fatigues stepped forward and offered his hand. It was a meeting that was going to transform my life beyond all recognition. I didn't know it right at that moment, but I had found my calling. My life was about to go helter-skelter.

14

The hospital staff gave me the mirror. I took it in my left hand because I couldn't bend my right, the tissue around the elbow joint having ossified into a solid mass and it stuck out like I was giving the Hitler salute. It's called myositis, they told me, but sorting that out was a long way down the list of priorities.

I barely had a world to collapse, but what was left of it fell inwards on me the moment I took the mirror in my bandaged mitt and quickly angled it towards me – to get it over and done with, face up to it like a man. It did feel like an implosion, the gravitational pull of the black hole sucking my star into a giant darkness in the blink of an eye. Actually, I didn't have a blinking eyelid at the time, but the hit to my soul was instantaneous. I'm not exaggerating for dramatic effect. It was a huge physical sensation, this gravity annihilating all hope, extinguishing the faint glimmers of light I had started to see in my future. The hunter in me, desperately fighting for a route out of the woods, sat down in a heap and gave up the search.

I was a hideous sight, the Elephant Man after falling asleep under a high-powered sunlamp. The skin all over was a livid red, raw and ravaged by flame and scalpel – or carpentry plane or whatever the hell they used. Mum had told me that Shelley and his team had done an amazing job on me. Really? I'd hate to see the job they screwed up. They might just as well have gone at it with a potato peeler and a garden fork. It takes time to heal, of course – and Shelley's team did do sensational work in a very long and delicate operation, particularly around the eyes, all that debriding, harvesting, grafting, slicing, cutting and pasting. But an urgency to high-five the surgery team was not my first reaction on looking at my mutilated face, the sight made all the worse by the rest of the damage: no hair, no eyebrows, stumps for ears, eyes staring back at me like a monkfish. It was grotesque.

A lot of people don't like their appearance but I felt physically sick looking at mine. It was truly disgusting. I was truly disgusting. I dropped the mirror and stared at the ceiling. Over the previous days a small bud of hope had sprouted in me. I had started plotting ways to squeeze some purpose out of the future. I would do a marathon, even if it took all day on my hands and knees. I could do charity work. I could set up an adventure tourism company. The hope was rising. But it took just one look in that mirror to lop that little bud, cauterise the spur and kill all hope of growth. You need light to grow and my light had been well and truly snuffed. *Fuck that for a life.* And I closed my eyes and slid back into the darkness.

Not long after, I went into septic shock. I couldn't have cared less. Drifting in and out, I was aware there was a major panic on before it went critical and I was put deep under again. I had continued to be dogged by septic episodes since my return to the UK. On flesh so hospitable and inviting as mine it was impossible to keep the MRSA and other invasive infections at bay, the open wounds guarded by an immune system so feeble and ingratiating to such insistent bacterial visitors. A steady flow of strong antibiotics flowed through my circulation, but it was never enough. It didn't help that they had discovered in Orlando that I reacted badly to Colistin, an antibiotic of last resort to multi-drug resistant infections.

The crisis came on very quickly, not long before Christmas. I remember my temperature sky-rocketing, getting the shivers and shakes, my breathing rapid and laboured, the night nurse erupting into frantic activity. Mum told me afterwards she was at her friend Malcolm's and was just settling down for the night on the sofa when she got the call on her mobile from the nurse. Malcolm told her she'd be better off getting a good sleep in first then, first thing in the morning, head down refreshed for what sounded like a long day. Had it been Orlando, with all their staff and resources, Mum may have left it and taken Malcolm's advice. But the Broomfield and NHS were not blessed with such riches, excellent use that they made with what they had. Mum waited until Malcom had gone upstairs then slipped out and belted down the down M1, around the M25 and up the A12 to Chelmsford. The journey ordinarily took her about 90 minutes, two hours in the rush, but she was in the hospital car park within the hour. There's no way the nurse would have called unless she was freaked out and thought she was going to lose me. Why else call the mother at midnight and get her to drive 75 miles?

Mum said I was hot to the touch even through the bandages. The night duty doctor, running here and there, sanctioned an intravenous infusion of super-antibiotics. The nurse brought in a trolley laden with bags of ice and she and Mum set about packing me like a lobster in a fishmonger's window display. I had bags under my arms, across my chest, over and around my groin and under my back. The nurse barely left my side the first night, in the end ordering Mum to go and get her head down. For two nights and two days my temperature raged, my body battling the eruption of infection. My kidneys went again and I was hooked up to a dialysis machine. Later, Mum told me she genuinely feared for me over that 48 hours. I didn't tell her that, had I been conscious, I would have told them to forget it, let nature take its course.

15

I was 25 years old when I enrolled at UEA in 2000, a mature student. I'd been in the police for three years and travelled around the world twice. I wasn't like most undergraduates and I had no interest in sitting around every weekend in the Students' Union smoking roll-ups, drinking cut-price lagers and mulling whether to have chilli sauce or garlic mayo on my kebab. Every now and then, sure, but not as a pastime. Nor did I join the Officer Training Corps because I was a guns 'n' ammo nut. I had no interest in that macho stuff, wearing combats as casuals, going on a paintball weekend and coming back thinking you're Rambo. I joined the OTC because a) they paid you to do it and I needed funds, b) I wanted to dodge the bars and clubs at the weekend, c) I had grown to respect and enjoy my fitness. Joining the OTC took down three birds with one stone.

Cambridge University OTC is one of the best in the country, its history dating to the Napoleonic Wars. The rigorous entry trials weed out the half-hearted. The first year was basic training Military Training Qualification (MTQ) Level One, pretty well the same course you complete if you join a regular army regiment, learning: leadership, drill, combat first aid, weapon handling, foot patrolling, fieldcraft, platoon level tactics, comms skills, map reading, riot control, fitness. The drills and exercises took place at the weekends and occasional evenings up in bases and training areas in Cambridgeshire. The training was no more than the basics but I loved it and they even paid for my train fares down from Norwich, on top of a small amount of beer money.

The recruitment literature for the Cambridge OTC was at pains to stress that 'university study is always a student's priority. All training is designed around your academic calendar.' I must have missed or skim-read that paragraph.

I enjoyed my time on the UEA campus in Norwich, occasionally joining the other students at the subsidised Union bar to down a few 'turbo-shandies' (a strong alcopop mixed with a half of cider and blackcurrant cordial). But only occasionally – because it was the OTC that dominated my student days.

Except when we were away on exercise, every weekend I made the one-hour fifteen-minute train journey down to Cambridge and jogged the one-and-a-half miles out to the OTC base. Situated on the perimeter of the city airport, right at the end of the runway, the grounds include a large lake and acres of land for fitness and field training.

The OTC is part of the Army Reserve and its principal aim is to train up and encourage students to serve in the Regular or Territorial Army, but there is no obligation to join up full-time after graduation. The cadets perform many of the challenges that trainee officers must pass in the full-blown course at Sandhurst, but they do it piecemeal, discipline by discipline, from basic soldiering and weapon-handling through to leadership skills and fieldcraft.

The OTC has a great social life too and, after a day's training, the cadets often enjoyed a hard-earned night at the bar or around the barbeque. I was having just as much fun as I would back in Norwich, but I was growing as a person too, pushing myself and learning new skills. Some students joined theatre groups or sports clubs, but for me, so active and driven since my wayward teenage years, the OTC was the place to get all the kicks and satisfaction my restless nature craved. The best mates I made at uni were fellow cadets and we ended up sharing a house together.

For the most committed, like me, the OTC dominated the university holiday periods too, offering and funding training programmes all over the world. At the end of my first year, I won a scholarship and joined two-dozen others from the wider OTC network at a huge US Army training camp in Fort Lewis, near Seattle. It was part of an exchange programme lasting six weeks and the American end of it was run by instructors from the US Special Forces and US Rangers. It was general military training, but it was tough, just how I was starting to like it: being pushed as hard and far as I could go. It was my first true taste of army life and, buoyed by the enthusiasm of my American hosts, I found it truly inspiring. The exercises took place in the beautiful setting of the Cascade Mountains, the course finishing there with a gruelling march in full kit over several days and nights. In the graduation ceremony at the end, watching the US cadets I had befriended pass out as commissioned officers was a moving experience – and a seed had been planted in my own mind.

Every holidays during my time at UEA, I took part in some form of adventure training at an exotic location overseas – and a few, on the quiet, during term time too. There were half-a-dozen expeditions to Norway, two climbing trips, the Fort Lewis exercise, two biathlons in Austria and a diving expedition to Egypt. A couple of years after leaving it, big new experiences under my belt, I would still tell you the OTC was 'the best club in the world' and had 'transformed my life'. The OTC had given me experiences I could never have dreamed of affording on my shoestring student budget; it had brought me the gift of many friendships, it had given me multiple career options. Above all, it had helped to turn the boy into a man.

I was lucky too with my branch of the corps. The Cambridge outfit had a long history of producing high-calibre cadets. Being comprised mainly of Cambridge University undergraduates, the recruits tend to be highly intelligent as well as robust and resourceful. Many of them headed to Sandhurst after their studies to finish off what they had started but, some, like me, took one of the short courses on offer there while still an undergraduate.

Eager to get on in my first year, maybe impress the seniors and instructors by my willing, I was foolish enough to try for a place on the Cambridge team for the Cambrian Patrol, the notorious international military exercise. This involves teams of eight trying to cover a 40-mile course in under 48 hours while completing a variety of military manoeuvres and tests. It sounds straightforward enough, but listening to veterans of it, I was given to understand that I would never previously have pushed myself anywhere near the limits of endurance that it demands. The Black Mountains and the Brecon Beacons, and the swampland skirting the high ground, provide the unforgiving terrain. In mid-autumn, the Welsh weather plays its part to make the experience as unpleasant as possible. It would be hard enough in perfect conditions.

Each year, teams fly in from military units around the world to test their endurance and skill levels. Of the 60 to 100 units that take part, between a half and a third do not complete the course, each team being only as strong as its weakest member. The Royal Marines send teams but the SAS decline for fear, so they say, that they would get beaten. The more prosaic truth is that they are too busy doing the day job.

The trials for the Cambrian took place early on in the autumn term, and I had barely set a new boot inside the OTC door when I put my hand up for a slot on the team. *No harm in giving it a shot*, I thought, *get a taste of it for another year maybe.* Two dozen of us cadets went up for the trials and at the end of the weekend I was amazed to learn I had been selected. I was, if nothing else, naturally fit and, light but wiry strong, I had a good physique for that type of challenge. Most of the Cambridge team had already competed in the Cambrian and my great fear was that I would let them down. I went straight into an intensive training programme. The Patrol was just six weeks away.

My nerves on the day were not helped by the atrocious weather conditions crashing in off the Atlantic. We jogged away from the start line, full-weight Bergen pack on the back, already soaked to the skin. We quick-marched day and night, up mountains and through bogs, squelching and tripping over a minefield of 'baby heads', the mounds of thick sedge that punctuate that bastard-grim terrain.

I had read the stories about soldiers of the Great War sleeping as they marched and thought it a bullshit exaggeration, a myth. But the cynical misgivings were dispelled when, a day in, we hit a tarmacked lane and I went into automaton sleep mode. When I woke up I was at a rendezvous point with a sergeant-major type bellowing hell into my ear.

I loved the musketeer camaraderie of it, all for one and one for all, each member dropping back to big up the guy struggling in the rear. Under the strain, each of our characters began to reveal themselves, our strengths shining out and our weaknesses laid bare. It was a pleasant slow-burn surprise to discover that I had as much stamina and will power as anyone, and I soon found myself in the role of cheerleader-in-chief. Drained to the marrow, yes, but I learned I had that little extra spare capacity to give motivation to others. I was relieved not to screw it up for the rest and, as the most junior, be able to make a positive contribution to the effort.

The survival instinct helps to keep you moving. It was so goddam cold and we were so wet, we knew that if we were to stop, we'd be placing ourselves and our teammates in grave danger. Hypothermia is a killer and the back-up teams raced around in their trucks and jeeps to bring in those who had succumbed. It was easy to understand why the British Army train their elite troops in mid-Wales. They may not be the coldest – and certainly never the hottest – but in their own way the bogs and mountains of Cambria are as harsh as any environment on the planet. You are so drenched you may as well have jumped in a lake. Recruits have died up there. Hypothermia doesn't take long to dispatch you.

The only time we stopped was to eat, shit or form up at one of the rendezvous points to complete a skills tasks, such as ID'ing enemy vehicles in the form of full-size inflatable models away in the distance, or treating a fallen comrade – a roleplay soldier – for medivac from the battlefield. They want you to push your brain as well as your body. The aim of the Cambrian is to imitate real operational scenarios as faithfully as possible – and those who compete never complain about the lack of realism.

It was the most gruelling two days of my life so far but, in a perverse way, the happiest. It was, up till then, the greatest achievement of my life, no question. I had pushed himself way further than I could ever have imagined. Cambridge came third in an international field of elite units – an incredible achievement for a bunch of student amateurs – and I had played my part in that. At the debrief, the commander handed out the medals and made a speech that was part congratulation and, to the Brits in the room, part recruitment. If you got a kick out of that, he said, then have a serious think about Special Forces Selection for the SAS. If you can complete a Cambrian, you're in with a shout.

So I did think about it, all the way back to East Anglia, slumped at the rear of the minibus, my body an empty shell but my soul a balloon. Anyone can get fit, but not everyone can be strong – strong of heart and mind. I had just discovered I had hidden depths of strength. I was going to give Special Forces a crack. One day. First, I had to complete the degree course I had only just begun.

16

Unfortunately, I recovered from the especially nasty bout of sepsis and began a slow and embittered recovery. I was a horrible patient. I hated everyone including most of the underpaid, overworked nurses who looked after me every day. I hated them because I hated myself even more, I hated what was left of my life and I hated the thought of what lay ahead. I was in a great deal of physical pain too. That never encourages a sunny disposition. The nurses at the Chelmsford stepdown ward must have been hardened over the years by the experience of tending to patients in savage pain and profound despair. It must be tough, shift after shift, tending the hopeless, the helpless, the desperate, the ungrateful, the bad-tempered and the downright rude, covered in sick, shit, pus and piss. Maybe they only do it because they know it might be them lying there one day. They sure don't do it for the money and the opportunity of meeting charming people.

I displayed all those horrible qualities during my re-emergence into consciousness on that ward. I became a caricature of anger. But I didn't care. I didn't care about me, my feelings, so why should I care about others, their feelings? To hell with me, to hell with you, just about summed up my attitude. I was angry at the world and I took it out on everyone around me. No longer in a coma, the little loss adjustor in my head was able to assess the damage and he regretted having to inform me that my life was a write-off. *With no sell-on value, Mister Hull, I am sorry to have to notify you that you*

and your useless heap of body are destined for the scrapheap – that's a
shame because that's a decent bit of kit you had there once upon a time.

Before the accident, I would describe myself as a man of
action and independent outlook. I was always on the move,
engaged in activities and adventures or planning them. I never
asked others to do what I could do for myself. I struck out into the
world on my own. That self-reliance was embedded in my behaviour through the experiences of my teenage years. I had taken
that greed for action to extremes in my pursuit of the outdoor life
and a career in the Armed Forces. In my army career, I had passed
just about the highest tests of self-sufficiency and resourcefulness
a man can undertake.

It was therefore the cruellest torture to find myself utterly
immobilised, unable to perform even the simple tasks of feeding myself, washing myself, going to the toilet, reading a book,
plumping up my pillows, scratching my elbow, blowing my nose
or changing the TV channel. It was for this reason that I hated the
people helping me. It was a humiliation, an insult to my dignity
and the sense of self-worth I had built up over the years. Destroying my freedom to act on my own terms began destroying my
soul with indecent haste. Looking back, I am not sure which I
role I most pity: mine or that of the people looking after me.

Chirpy people were the worst. Chirpiness was a state of being,
an outlook on the world, from which it was impossible for me to
be further removed. I was the extreme opposite of chirpy. If you
googled synonyms for chirpy, the search engine would offer 'Jamie
Hull' as the antonym. If you were a chirpy soul, you entered my
cheerless sphere at your peril. People visiting the gravely infirm
have the notion that they must be upbeat, positive, optimistic –
chirpy, chirpy, cheep, cheep. The graver the problem, the higher
the chirp. My situation was extremely grave so I suffered a lot
of chirp.

As a world expert in receiving bedside visits, a word of advice: don't be fucking chirpy. Be morose, be downbeat, be negative. Only then will you be in full sympathy with the person you are visiting. Chirpy is a theatrical and insincere display of happiness; the patient can smell the bullshit coming off it as it makes its way down the corridor. Chirpy makes a patient feel even more miserable. The happiest visits I received were from friends who told me how crap their life was at that time, that their lives had gone wrong in one way or another – their job, their marriage, their health, whatever. I could relate to that. *Great, you're sad too!*

Tell me the weather had been awful and there'd be a little spike in my happiness levels. Tell me you'd lost your job and I might even smile. Tell me you'd come off your motorbike and shattered your leg – that would keep me going for the rest of the day. But come in and tell me you had an incredible skiing holiday in the Tyrol, got engaged to a beautiful girl and came home to find you'd been promoted, you'd get a little side-of-the-mouth smile off me. Then, after you'd gone, feeling chuffed you'd cheered up your old mate, I would sink into the darkest and bitterest of moods. Sorry, but that's the way it was.

The chirpiest people are always to be found on the television. If I had had a way of herding them all up, maybe with a special remote control device, driving them into a giant burial pit and setting fire to them, I would have done that with no more emotion than making myself a cup of tea. People on reality shows may not have been the chirpiest but they soon topped my imaginary shopping list of customised voodoo dolls. I'd stare at the screen, scowling and thinking: *You want some reality, come and sit in my bed, arsehole!* And then there was the daytime talk-show episode about living with a partner who snores ... boy, the burdens people have to carry, the crosses they bear.

If ever I was to become a professional torturer, and that was starting to look like an attractive career option from where I sat, I'd immobilise my victim and make them watch daytime chats on a continuous 24-hour loop with the volume really high. But if I *really* wanted to hurt them, or I was desperate to extract the required intelligence, I'd make them listen to *Steve Wright in the Afternoon* on the radio. Steve Wright, the king of chirp. I found it incredible – hated myself even more – that I had wasted so many hours of my life listening to that bubbly bastard. One of the few ways I found to cheer myself was to imagine myself punching his face all day long. A dayshift nurse who really hated me (take your pick) got wise to my loathing of the King of Chirp. One afternoon, after the nurse and I'd had an especially bad fallout, she put on Radio 2, turned up the volume and left me to stew for an hour. I'd had a lot of low moments since catching fire, but that was just about the worst. Sorry, Steve, you're a consummate professional, Britain's most listened-to disc jockey, you obviously mean well and you've got a lively little show going there. But I really hate you. Your chirp was the salt in my red raw wounds. Go fuck yourself.

After a time on the stepdown ward, my bile-yellow naso-gastric tube was removed and I no longer ate my meals through my nose. I was moved on to solids. 'Solids' struck me as a poor choice of word, its meaning bearing no resemblance to the reality of the stuff in the bowl. Sure, it's not quite as liquid as the stuff that went up my nostrils, but it was still very runny mush. Unable to use cutlery, the solids were fed to me on a little rubber spoon as used for babies fresh off the teet. This was a great indignity. I used to be adept at catching my own food in the wild and cooking it over a fire made from flint sparks. Now I was being told to 'Open wide, there's a good boy.' That's some fall from grace.

There was good reason why my solids had been pulver-ised into baby food. I used to throw it up, generally about five minutes after the nurse had finished spooning it in and it had been given the time to slide down my gullet into the opening of my very tender stomach. It was an undignified spectacle and experience, this opening wide for nursey, and it got worse when nursey, busy and exhausted always, came back in and saw the puke. Hands on hips in mock despair, she would say something like, 'Now Jamie, who's been a naughty boy again?' or 'Good heavens, what *are* we going to do with you?' She was trying to be gentle and forgiving, of course, but I was hoping I had kept back a bit of puke to land on her. *Come on, nursey, just a couple more steps this way.*

She'd begin the process of cleaning me up and changing my bed linen and, if necessary, any wound dressings that had taken a jet of spew. The only way to change my sheets, being unable to hop out of bed for the operation, was to be manhandled. This was always painful because much of my skin remained unhealed – the plastic surgeons harvesting as quick as the skin grew back on the donor sites. The nurse rolled me on to my side, me yelping and groaning, sometimes crying, and pulled out the sheets. The process was repeated on the other side and then again with the fresh sheets. This was another excellent form of torture to add to my list: humiliate the captive by asking him to open wide, feed him a few spoons of disgusting baby mush, trigger projectile puke, shove and roll blistered and peeled body until pain becomes intolerable.

It was the same with being washed, another monstrous indignity, painful and demeaning. God, I hated my daily wash. It all seemed so pointless when I was carpeted in MRSA. There was black mould all over me and when it was scraped and scrubbed off, it just came back. So, what was the point in washing me? If I can live with deadly infections of invasive bacteria, I can live with body odour. Shove your sponge. It was even more demeaning when, aged 32, it's your mother doing the washing, scrubbing behind what used to be your ears.

It had been over six months since I had walked. The last step I took was over the wing of a burning aircraft. Looking down, judging the time to go for it, flames hammering one side of me, the rubber soles of my hiking trainers melting and the buckskin suede uppers smoking. I remembered the peculiarity of that image, like something you see in a cartoon. I was as fit as anyone on the planet when I had my accident. That's not a boast, just a plain fact. I may not have been the fastest or the best over long distance, but I don't see how my general fitness levels can have been any higher. I was about to go on operational deployment. I needed to be in perfect condition and I was. If you woke me one morning and told me I had to run a marathon, even back-to-back marathons, I'd put on my trainers and go do it. I'd be struggling at the end, of course, because that's what happens at the end of marathons. No human body feels fresh as a daisy after it's been run for 26 miles. But I'd do it for you, no sweat.

Now, lying in Chelmsford, if there was a fire and all the nurses had fled from my room (high probability – they needed no second invitation), I would not have made it halfway to the door even on my hands and knees. That's because I had no muscles. They had wasted to nothing. I was skin and bone (burned and grafted skin) with a bit of charred tissue and distorted ligament here and there. So, the physio began in earnest. Before I could walk, I first had to learn to sit. Just like a baby graduating to infancy. The muscles in my abdomen no longer existed. I had the posture of a sack of shit.

While I was in my coma, others were doing my exercise for me. In Chelmsford, as in Orlando, physiotherapists came twice a day to bend and twist my moving parts and massage what they could of the fleshier areas. This was to stop the joints from seizing up, keep the blood circulation flowing and strengthen my wasting muscles. There is medical evidence showing that 'touch' might help the healing process too. Physios will often talk to the coma patient as they work the body. They make a strong argument that this multisensory communication is absorbed by the brain and accelerates recovery.

Soon after my transfer to the stepdown, the head of my bed was raised periodically and I was propped up against a bank of pillows. This was not for my comfort. It was for me to learn to sit, to build up my core stomach and back muscles and encourage greater movement of my limbs. Sitting up, you are more likely to reach out for an object than if you are flat on your back. All movement, any movement was to be encouraged, but the lower half of me was in no mood for exercise. My groin muscles had gone. Raising a knee was not an option anyhow because my legs were stiff with dressings and bandages from the constant debriding, grafting and harvesting.

The plastic surgeons – a first-class outfit – were tireless in their efforts to get skin on me: my own skin, the skin of the dead and the skin of pigs. (They only told me about the pigs much later to spare my feelings and, I suspect, to stop me throwing an accusing finger at the more hateful nurses). The sooner they got some cover on my crappy infected flesh the better for everyone. The better for me, to put an end to the recurring bouts of sepsis; the better for the nurses and my mum – they spent hours and hours, week after week, changing my dressings – and the better for the hospital. From the day of my admission, I had been attracting every form of invasive infection – MRSA, C. difficile, pseudomonas, name your bacteria or fungi and I had it. I was soon a major cause for concern, and not just for my own well-being.

Like all NHS hospitals, Chelmsford had a serious MRSA crisis at the time, so radical cleansing regimes were being introduced and the infection police were on the prowl. They certainly didn't need any sly tip-offs from informers to uncover my crimes of bacteria. There was no hiding them. I was an infection disco, a huge unlicensed bacterial rave and a blessed nuisance to the wider community. The sooner – infection-wise – I was shut down, the happier the neighbourhood and the authorities were going to be.

Once I had mastered the basics of sitting, I advanced to the challenge of standing. The exercise was known as 'sit-to-stand', and it would be simple enough, you'd think, to swing out my legs, drop them to the floor and lean against the side of the bed. I never cried during any of the gruelling exercises and courses I undertook with the army, but I did cry during these sit-to-stand manoeuvres. It took the most incredible effort and caused an extraordinary amount of pain and panic. I was so weak and dizzy from meds, anaemia and poor circulation that each time I made this effort to stand I came close to fainting, my trembling legs always just about to give way at the knees.

I had physios either side poised to hook their arms under my armpits if I buckled, and tears poured down my cheeks, the salt in the wounds making a minor contribution to the pain. This tiny action, leaning against my bed, was all I could manage for about two weeks. When the ordeal was over and I returned to the comfort of my mattress and pillows, I fell straight into a deep sleep, shattered by the expenditure of mental, physical and emotional energy. Again, it was the humiliation as much as the pain and frustration that was getting to me. I had never leaned on anyone for anything in my life. Now I couldn't even stand up without help.

From sitting to standing to my first baby steps. I approached the prospect of walking with the same mindset that I had taken into the Cambrian Patrol and army selection tests. I had to steel myself for the challenge and I was half nervous, half excited. I knew it was going to be excruciatingly painful and difficult, but I was bloody well going to do it. I knew from my past challenges that if I could get myself over the line, then the sense of achievement was going to be enormous.

The line, in the first instances, was the end of the bed. I looked down at it as I once looked up at Pen-y-Fan, a mountain in the Brecon Beacons. With my flesh so raw still, the physios could not risk having to seize me if I collapsed, so I was placed in a special walking harness that gave me a modicum of support and acted as a safety net when I fell.

It was a weird feeling to be upright. It was not a sensation I had experienced since standing on the wing of my burning aircraft. All my experience of the world since then had come in the horizontal position. That's odder than it may sound. It was strange too how so rudimentary an action as putting one foot in front of another should feel like a huge and daring adventure, offering the same thrills and fears of any of the extreme sports I used to practise. My adrenal levels had been dangerously low since the accident, but they rose sharply when I stood there filling my lungs, stabbing out breaths, closed my eyes and finally found the courage to go for it and throw out a foot.

One of the reasons, I was to discover, that I found this daily effort so tough was because I no longer had any muscles in my shins. They had been cleared out in Orlando, I was told eventually, in order to prevent my legs being amputated. There was just the fibula bone there now with a poor excuse for some skin slapped on top and periodically carpeted with infection. My other muscles, such as they existed at the time, were having to be taught to take the load. I was learning to walk for the second time in my life.

After a week of excursions to the end of my bed, I began to venture further afield to more exotic locations. Like the wall and the door. This was all leading up to the greatest mission of all – the journey to the *en-suite* bathroom. The toilet, for those backing my voyage of discovery, was the principal goal of my expedition. Captain Cook went to Australia and New Zealand, Christopher Columbus to the Americas, Neil Armstrong to the moon. Jamie Hull went to the toilet.

It may not have been going out live around the world, but I for one was very excited about my voyage into the unknown. I couldn't wait for the day I could wipe my own arse again. Or piss into a porcelain bowl and no longer have to contort myself like Houdini under the sheet to relieve myself into a recycled cardboard eggbox. Sticking close to land, I navigated along the shoals of my bed, negotiating a route between the twin hazards of my portable overbed table and the visitor's armchair. Taking a deep breath, I launched myself (in my harness) into the wide open, uncharted spaces of the lino flooring, a vast expanse of two metres, and hurled myself towards the bathroom door, hitting speeds of up to 0.5 miles an hour at times in the rush to accomplish my historic goal.

I made it! I was panting and sweating but I did it! Everyone was delighted. *He made it!* There was cheering and, had there been hats to hand, I am sure they would have been thrown into the air. In the event, my first unaided shit was not the great experience I had looked forward to with so much excitement. Sure, getting there was a great achievement, but the crouching was agonising, my skin stretching and cracking like a family pack of crisps. The shit itself was a disappointing runny texture and wiping my arse with my mangled left hand was an episode of dark comedy. Try it at home – a gardening glove will suffice for bandages. I wonder if Neil Armstrong felt the same when he leaped from Apollo 11's lunar lander and hit the moondust. *So, that's it, eh?* Slowly I made my way back to where I had launched off all that time ago, to home sweet home, my bed, and I plunged into the deepest of sleeps, my little place in history assured.

If the toilet trip was a minor disappointment, the expedition to the bath was a full-blown nightmare, a voyage equivalent to rounding Cape Horn in a force 10. It was a journey I had to make many times. By some distance, this event, which took place every other day, ranks as one of the most terrible experiences of my life. Once the relief had worn off after one bath (that is, as soon as I had woken up after the horror of the last), I began to dread the prospect of the next one.

The nurses/secret police marched into my room that first time. All my wound dressings were removed and I shuddered with cold. The air wasn't cold at all, it was room temperature, but I couldn't have felt colder if I had been dumped on an icefloe. They wheeled me down the corridor to a bathroom in some sort of hoisting contraption and I was lowered into the deep tub like a submersible from an exploration ship. The lukewarm water was lovely, the first pleasurable sensation on my skin I had felt since I had walked out on that beautiful summer morning and looked up into the Florida sunshine. I closed my eyes and sighed. 'Ah, lovely, can I have one of these every day?'

Then the nurses went to work with their sponges. I howled. It was as if I was on fire again. They went at the wounds with rapid circular motions, trying to get it over and done with, but to get the infection off me they had to be thorough and brutal on my open wounds. I was roaring, 'Stop! Stop! Please fucking stop!' I have made dark jokes about torture, but this was the closest I have come to that dreadful experience. Truly, there cannot be many more effective ways of one human being inflicting pain on another. It took no more than three or four minutes but by the time they were done and the hoist winched me out of the warm water, I was sobbing and shaking, an Arctic wind gripping my scoured, bleeding skin.

After a few more weeks, my muscles had strengthened sufficiently and I advanced to a shower. No event in my life was quick and straightforward. The most insignificant task – pissing, eating, washing – was an ordeal and a major logistical operation. My first shower since the morning of 19 August 2007 was no different.

After witnessing my bath, Mum had learned to leave the room and head for a coffee at washing time. She couldn't bear to watch her son being savagely assaulted. It was meant kindly, of course, but it was still a savage assault, just without the intention to wound or maim. If you could prove intention in a court of law, the nurses/secret police could get up to ten years for that degree of barbarity. There was a different instrument of torture for the shower, a kind of child's mobile swing, me parked naked on the seat below the frame. There also a big cylinder on a trolley containing Entonox, an inhaled gas (50 per cent nitrous oxide, 50 per cent oxygen) used as pain medication in childbirth, trauma and end-of-life care. It is used in conjunction with other analgesics and, as always, I was coursing with my regular doses of morphine, ibuprofen, paracetamol and tramadol hydrochloride.

The nurses donned long plastic aprons, latex gloves, shower caps, face masks and clogs, looking every inch like mortuary technicians about to conduct an autopsy. One of them turned on the shower, adjusting the temperature, and the room filled with a pleasant gentle mist. The other helped me to put the tube into my mouth and I took a deep draught of happy gas. The little high was only momentary.

I was wheeled under the cascading water, and the sensation was both pleasure and pain, the pleasure coming from the warmth of soothing water running down my body, the pain from the rods of it that cascaded into my back like hailstones. But it was ecstasy, relative to what followed.

The nurses took up position, plunged their sponges into the bucket of antiseptic water and went at me like they were sanding a wall. It can't have been a pleasant experience for them – unless they were sadists – because I didn't stop hollering and crying from the first minute to the fifth and last. I was so busy screaming, gasping and choking on my tears I was barely able to get the happy gas tube into my mouth. When I did, I chuffed on it like I was running up a hill, pumping it in with short rapid breaths, but the effect of it was barely noticeable. Nothing short of a full coma can alleviate the pain of being cheese-grated. That's an accurate description of it. I cannot imagine how a grater, forcefully applied up and down my open wounds, can have been any less excruciating. It's the same nerve endings being shredded after all. When it was over, I sat head over my knees, chest heaving, gagging on my tears, watching my fluids, pus and blood, swirling around the tiled floor and down the plughole, the perfect metaphor for my life.

I hated Chelmsford, every conscious second of my three-and-a-half months there. The plastic surgeons, led by Peter Dziewulski and Odhran Shelley, were top drawer and they and their team did incredible work in patching me up. The treatment and care in the intensive care unit was first class too, so Mum told me, as good as I'd get anywhere in the UK. Not in the same league of quality as Orlando, but Orlando was as good as anywhere in the world.

That's the difference between private treatment and a free publicly funded service. The NHS is a remarkable institution, but its resources are limited. They work miracles with what they are given. If you need emergency treatment or intensive care, you will get world-class service in Britain. But if your life's no longer in immediate danger, the standards drop off sharply.

That is not a criticism of the people who cared for me. You won't find me moaning about people who devote their lives to the care of others. Most of the nurses were great, one or two lovely, but one or two were genuinely heartless and I hate them now as I hated them then. (There are over 250,00 nurses in the NHS and, by the laws of statistics, you are always going to get a couple of bastards.) That was my experience anyhow – an experience intensified by the re-emergence into consciousness and the terrible realisation of my condition, the extreme and never-ending pain, the frustrations of being utterly dependent on others and a depression that was deepening by the day.

I couldn't get shot of Chelmsford fast enough. Luckily, they wanted shot of me even more urgently.

17

I was studying all four main Scandinavian languages at UEA, majoring in Norwegian because of an old family connection and a deep-rooted curiosity about the Land of the Midnight Sun. Mum was born Kristensen, her mother having married a Norwegian soldier based in Scotland during the war. Always curious about my distant heritage, in September 2001, I was excited to fly out to spend a year living among the native speakers. Most foreign students head to the bright lights of Bergen or Tromsø, but I went inland, deep inland, into the remote, thinly populated wilderness of Sogn og Fjordane. There were bright lights – a scattering at least – but they tended to be turned off by ten o'clock. Going to Sogn og Fjordane was my tutor's idea and I will always be grateful to her for the wonderful experiences I enjoyed there. She had come to understand my weakness for the outdoors, my relish for a physical challenge. Sogn og Fjordane did not disappoint.

There was little formal studying out there. All the learning was achieved simply by living among Norwegians, absorbing and talking their language. The locals were reluctant or unable to speak English and so there was no skiving the task and I learned fast. No surprises, I spent most of the year outdoors, making the most of every one of the five or six hours of daylight in the winter months. To be honest, there aren't many indoors diversions in deepest Norway. All the fun's out in the cold air. As soon as the snows arrived, and they weren't long in coming, I took up skiing – 'back country' skiing up in the mountains and Nordic, or cross-country, skiing down on the flat. I took to it like a penguin, my high fitness levels allowing me to make rapid progress because, in this type of skiing, unlike Alpine, you have to create your own locomotion. I spent entire days deep in the wooded mountains, a world as far from the suffocating town life of Leighton Buzzard as could be imagined.

They were happy days, gruelling and hazardous sure, but as happy as any I could remember. It was my first experience of true mountain life and I savoured the same freedom, remoteness and enchanting otherworldliness I had found in scuba diving. The mountains, like the sea, offered a refuge, an escape. There was danger and adventure. I had to push myself hard, take risks, and the more I chased the adrenaline, the more I craved it.

Unable these days to resist a bigger challenge, I went a step further and blagged my way into the local Mountain Rescue team who were always happy to receive fresh volunteers and, in this instance, curious to have the 'crazy Englishman' in their number, for variety and entertainment if nothing else. They taught me all the skills – how to survive in the open, how to ski in the most difficult and remote areas, and how to rescue people.

My enthusiasm got the better of my judgement only once when, during an avalanche rescue exercise, not wanting to be thought cowardly, I volunteered to be buried alive. Dumb move. Discretion, I should have remembered, is always the better part of valour. It was, I must confess, the most frightening experience of my life – and I suffered nightmares for weeks afterwards. They dug me in nice and deep, and I lay in a tiny cocoon with just enough air to keep me alive. I was only down there for two or three minutes but it felt like an hour and I was in near-panic mode when they finally dug down to release me. It did genuinely feel like coming back from the dead.

I loved the skiing so much I was out all the time and became so proficient at it that, on my return with a fistful of certificates, the OTC commander in Cambridge had me trained up as a full instructor for the British Armed Forces. I needed no persuasion, and in my third year at UEA I made several returns to Norway, this time to the Hardangervidda plateau region. By the end of that winter I had qualified as a JSSI – a Joint Services Ski Instructor – and an STL, a mountain skiing tour leader. Putting my new skills to use, for the next two years I was tasked with running training expeditions for OTC troops in the Austrian Alps. Always up for the next challenge, I took up biathlons and was soon representing the British Army team in international competitions.

In the dark days of the deep Norwegian winter, there was never enough daylight to satisfy my voracious appetite for outdoor activity. I was getting restless, like a polar bear in the zoo, pacing back and forth. Stomping away on the treadmill kept up my fitness levels but it provided no thrills, just the sweat and the satisfaction of staying in shape. The worst that could happen in the gym was to go too fast and fall off – and where was the thrill in that? I overcame that mounting problem standing at my bedroom window one afternoon watching the gloom envelope the fjord. Before me lay the Sognefjord, the King of Fjords, the largest and deepest in Norway, its shores flanked by steepling cliffs rising to 1,000 metres. Running 130 miles inland from the ocean, for most of its length Sognefjord is over a kilometre deep. In Sogndal, far from the flow of the open seas, thick ice covered its surface. But there was plenty of water beneath. Problem solved. I'd go diving!

It is one of the golden rules of scuba diving that you should never go out alone. You need a buddy. Diving is a dangerous business. There are a hundred ways to die. When a beginner diver takes his PADI Open Water certificate, he is effectively learning how to avoid dying. On my travels, I had learned some of the skills and techniques of self-reliant – or 'independent' – diving, but without back-up on hand it is always a doubly hazardous enterprise, no matter how experienced. The danger doubles again when solo diving is undertaken at night and the diver cannot tell the difference between up and down, when you cannot see the surface even in shallow depths. In the ice-bound, pitch-black depths of Norway's deepest fjord, there are also increased risks of cramp and 'cold incapacitation' when blood shifts to the body's core to protect the organs, muscles lose power and the limbs become heavy.

I knew all this, but it wasn't going to stop me having an adventure and pushing myself to the limit – or rather, to the depths. Danger – great! It was a sight new to the locals and they watched with a mixture of amusement, astonishment and anxiety as 'their crazy Englishman', every other day or so, took to waddling down the wooden jetty opposite the school in his dive suit. The ice was solid and I smashed away at it with bricks and a hammer to create a hole large enough to fit a human body. I dropped a weighted rope into the depths and, after running through the equipment checks, strapped my big Russian Kowalski dive light to my wrist and, holding my mask in place, hopped off the jetty. Just like that – and the last sound I heard was the locals gasping before I disappeared under.

The first few dives, the locals waited anxiously for my return – often I'd be down there for almost an hour, diving as deep as 30 metres, the recommended maximum. All the time, I was aware that if I developed a problem with the regulator, I was finished. I had no buddy to come to my rescue and let me share his air. If I shot to the surface from depth, I'd likely die from decompression sickness – the bends – or at the very least suffer serious long-term damage. One malfunction and I would sink the kilometre to the

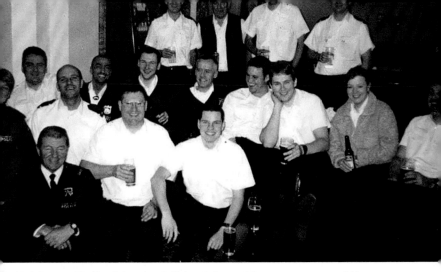

PC 1137 Hull, celebrating 'off-duty' time with a strong team – fellow Thames Valley Police Officers, Milton Keynes Station, October 1999

Travelling in style, courtesy of a British Army '4-tonner' truck, Africa, 2006

Somewhere very cold, the Arctic, 2007

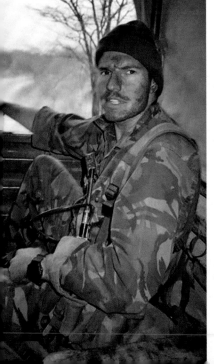

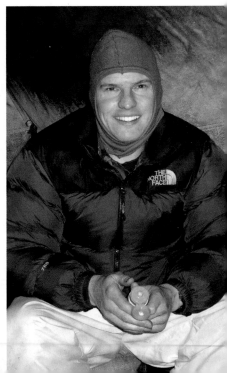

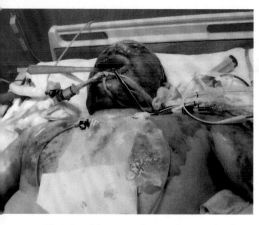

The shocking transformation my body went through in the first 24 hours post-burns trauma, ICU, Florida, USA, 19 August 2007

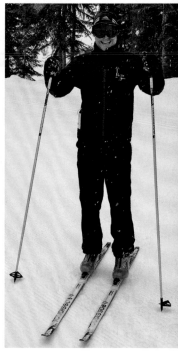

Nordic skiing with Help for Heroes, Vancouver, 2012

Winter Biathlon with Help for Heroes, Vancouver, 2012

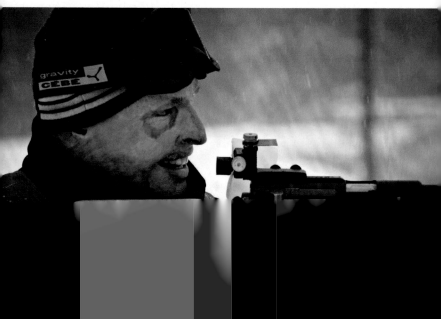

Testing my VO$_2$ max output in the lab at Cardiff University prior to the Race Across America in 2012 with Help for Heroes

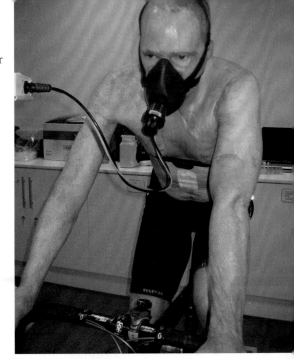

Leading an expedition in Africa, 2012

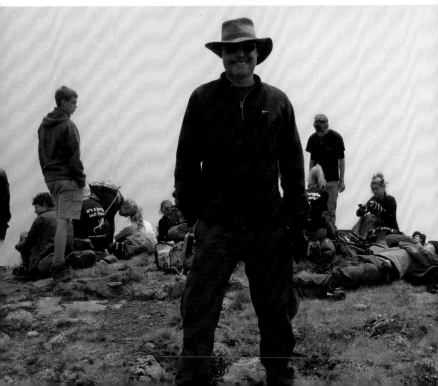

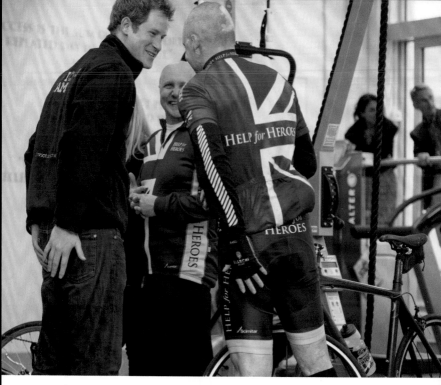

At the Invictus Games 2014 launch event at Tedworth House, emphasising the need for padded cycling shorts to Prince Harry

Standing tall with fellow burns survivors – all members of The Guinea Pig Club – in York, 2014

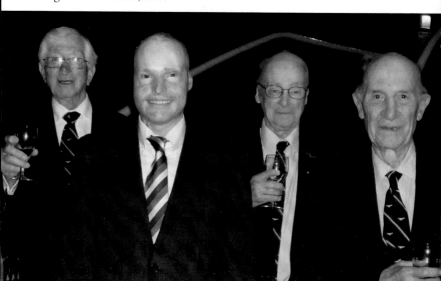

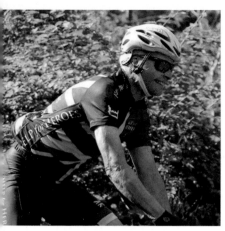

One of my greatest joys, cycling for
Help for Heroes, Paris to London, 2015

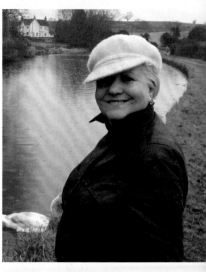

My mother
Shirley, enjoying
the great outdoors,
England, 2016

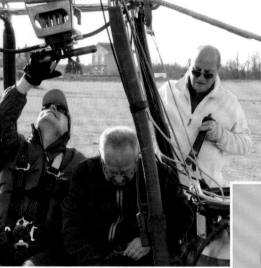

Piloting a hot air balloon
in Italy, 2016

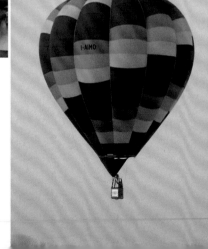

My first solo balloon
flight, Italy, 2016

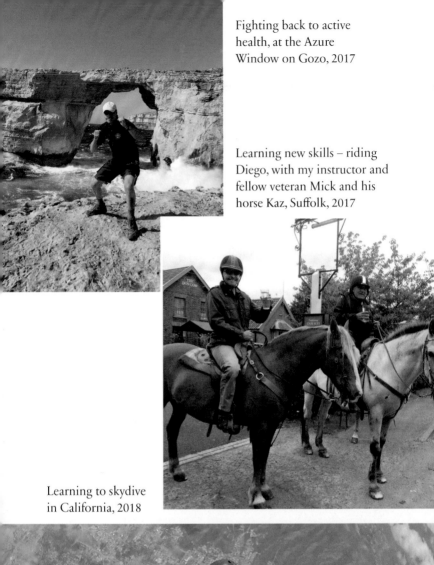

Fighting back to active health, at the Azure Window on Gozo, 2017

Learning new skills – riding Diego, with my instructor and fellow veteran Mick and his horse Kaz, Suffolk, 2017

Learning to skydive in California, 2018

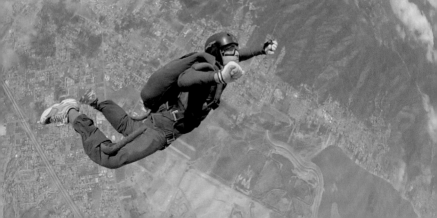

The new me, modelling T-shirts for Debenhams and Help for Heroes, London, 2018

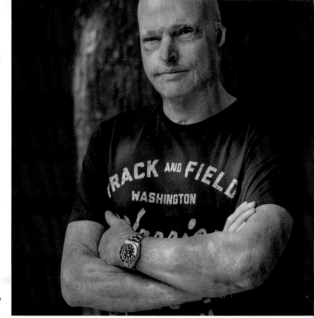

Teaching veterans to dive, the Red Sea, Egypt, 2019

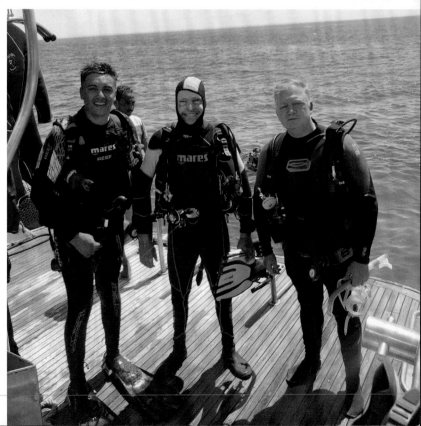

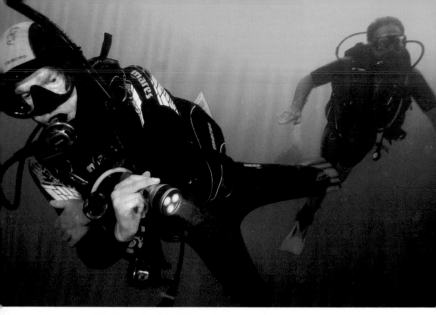

Diving with the injured, Djibouti, January 2020

Putting my best foot forward for The London Gala Ball, February 2020
– courtesy of Viktoriya Wilton, Inspiration to Dance

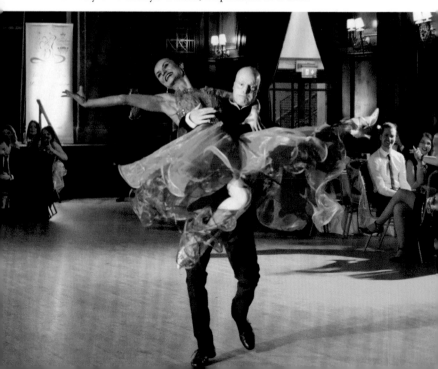

fjord floor, weighed down by my tank and kit, my neoprene-wrapped remains to lie undisturbed for the rest of time. It was a major risk but a major thrill too – and I couldn't resist it.

On the early dives, I'd pop back up through a hole like a seal to discover a knot of locals clapping and smiling in relief. Soon, local curiosity turned into genuine interest – perhaps fuelled by the long, dark evenings of a Norwegian winter when there is little to do but read, watch television or go to bed. So I began to give diving lessons, earning myself a few extra kroner to pay for the odd overpriced beer in one of the town's two bars.

Other than to sleep or sit and eat, I barely stopped moving for the entire nine months in Norway. I returned from Norway, feeling another foot taller, the horizons of my world stretched that much further again. And I could speak Norwegian! How many non-Norwegians can say that? My fluency would probably be of very little use in my life, but so what? It was a trophy and learning a new language is great for the brain muscles. My world was expanding like a new solar system. Leighton Buzzard was now just a very small pinprick on the map.

18

I was discharged from Chelmsford on 21 February 2008, meaning I was considered well enough to go home. Desperate as I was to leave, that came as a major surprise to me. Mum had been pushing for a transfer to Stoke Mandeville, a 25-minute hop from her house in Leighton Buzzard. The daily roundtrip of three to four hours was exhausting her, especially in the dark months of winter when the days were at their shortest and the weather at its most foul. At Chelmsford, there was no free, charitable accommodation as there was in Orlando with Hubbard House. That had been the most incredible blessing for her. Without Hubbard House, she would somehow have had to raise thousands of dollars for accommodation and living expenses to be at my side and consult with my medical team every day. Back in the UK, she could not afford to stay in a B&B. No longer in work, her funds were very limited so she had to shuttle back and forth in the car. That's not a complaint, just a bare fact. The charity SSAFA (Soldiers, Sailors, Airmen and Families Association) is a national treasure and when they came to the rescue and funded some nights for Mum in a B&B, she wept with relief and gratitude.

Stoke Mandeville was one of the best hospitals in the country and it had a very good plastic surgery department. It was also my local hospital. In a system working correctly, I would have been transferred there in an ambulance shortly after I was taken out of intensive care. Why I wasn't is a mystery. You may well share my incredulity at how the events unfolded and how the decisions to let me go were reached. I tell it not to point fingers and seek out individuals to blame. It's not an attack on the NHS. It's just what happened. As in most cases when institutions fail, it's the system that is faulty, not the people working in it.

When the day came, in spite of the saturation of antibiotics, I remained plastered in MRSA and I had continued to suffer potentially lethal septic episodes. The brilliant plastic surgeons at Chelmsford had worked on me as a team of sculptors might go at a huge lump of clay or block of stone. Thanks to their skill, I was starting to take shape, my resemblance to the human form increasing by the week. But I was still an aesthetic mess, and the proof of that could be found on my discharge summary, which assessed my disabilities with a biro-ed circle around 'permanent', and more scrawled loops around 'locomotor' and 'aesthetic'.

Locomotor did not mean that my toy train set was malfunctioning; it meant I couldn't walk very well and had no use of my right arm owing to the ossification of my elbow, a development that had granted me ongoing membership of the Nazi Party until I was fit for the operations to fix it. It was fortunate that I was unable to get up and walk around Chelmsford town centre because it is highly likely I would have been arrested and charged with hate crimes.

With the help of a nurse or physiotherapist, for a week or so I had been able to shuffle a short distance along the corridor outside my room, but it was an exhausting effort. Ridiculous as it may sound coming from a soldier, it was scary too. At any moment I felt that my knees might give way and I'd crash to the floor, incurring a fresh set of injuries. I had support, but high-wire adventurers will tell you that walking a tightrope at 500 feet is scary even with a safety net in place.

On the day of my departure from Chelmsford, I was not so mobile that I could be walked out to Mum's car. A wheelchair was laid on for the event, as much for reasons of liability as comfort. A week earlier, in a trial run, a nurse took me to a nearby pub for an orange juice and lemonade. This acclimatisation exercise was a pointless and miserable experience, me being wheeled in and everyone trying not to stare at the freak in the room. As on that occasion, on my discharge day I was dressed in the worst my wardrobe had to offer, my *Little Britain* fashion line: baggy tracksuits, massive nightie of a T-shirt and big shapeless cardigan, all of it as loose as possible so as to fit over the bandages with as little pressure and friction as possible. It being cold, and me even colder, I had a big woolly hat over the dressings on my scalp and a pair of gloves borrowed from a giant. Not that I cared, but I looked like a model for Monster Munch crisps.

With some effort I was fitted into the back seat of Mum's maroon Toyota Corolla and, driving like she was 112 so that I wasn't thrown about, bashing my wounds, we snailed out of the car park and on to the A12. Staying in the slow lane the whole way there, as good as stationary, we crawled around half the M25 orbital and up the M1. On finally arriving back in the little cul-de-sac in Leighton Buzzard, Mum set about unpacking me and my belongings, comprised almost entirely of medications and dressings. Unable to get up the stairs of her two-bedroom terraced house – that was a challenge to be undertaken on the advanced module of my walking course – Mum had set up a camp bed for me in the sitting room, with an en-suite commode on one side of the bed and a little table on the other, the television turned to face me.

With large areas of my skin unhealed and the MRSA colonising faster than the British Empire in its Victorian heyday, the plan down the line was for a district nurse to come and clean the wounds and change my dressings. Mum had been trained to do this at Chelmsford – clean out the pus, dry the area, apply the cream, then gauze and bind – but it was a hard task to perform, inflicting such pain on her son. So, until I healed some more, the instruction was to drive to Stoke Mandeville three times a week and have a shower there while I was about it.

The plan lasted less than 24 hours. I was in a great deal of pain when I left Chelmsford and I could just about handle that. Mum is tough and resourceful, and she could just about handle the care. But I was dangerously unwell with all the infections forever invading me, and my body was not yet strong enough to launch a counterattack powerful enough to defeat them. I was desperate for the restoration of some normality in my life and being at home was a step in that direction. But I was in no state to be home-nursed. Everyone knew that.

I spent an uncomfortable night on a regular bed, low to the ground and lacking the gadgetry to raise me up and tip me out. Levering myself up to use the commode was a huge ordeal. My father came over in the morning and together we set out for Stoke Mandeville. The official purpose was to have my dressings changed and go through the admissions procedure as an outpatient. But I knew I wasn't coming home. It is not an overstatement to claim that I might well have died had we stuck it out and I stayed at my mother's. At best, I would I have been blue-lighted into intensive care with septic shock and, if the ambulance wasn't there fast enough, with multi-organ failure.

It was a bitterly cold morning. I was past shivering and into full shaking as my parents helped me across the car park at Stoke Mandeville, the longest distance I had covered since I had left the courtesy home and headed to the airfield that morning. The pneumatic doors at the hospital entrance hissed open but I could go no further and my father went off to track down a wheelchair. The nurse who greeted us took one look at me and made an instant effort to correct the look of shock on her face. She was called Sister Adele and I liked her from the moment she thrust out her hand, spread a lovely warm smile and quickly wheeled me out of the waiting area and into a side room. She knew – even without having to take off my bandages. She didn't say, *You look like a dead man warmed up*, but her face did.

She hurried out and hurried back in, snapping on her latex gloves, and set about unravelling my dressings. I liked that she made no effort to hide her revulsion at the state of my wounds and her outrage that I had been discharged. She sighed and tutted and shook her head, and I felt the tears welling up. I was no more than a piece of meat gone off and cast out. I had experienced the opposite of care. I had experienced rejection and it was all the more painful to take because I felt so physically vulnerable and my morale was so fragile. I felt that the greatest indignity had been served upon me, to go begging for help. In a civilised country, you shouldn't have to ask for it when you are in a state of extreme vulnerability.

My spirits rose in Adele's presence. She was old-school: no-nonsense, straight-talking but chock full of compassion and common decency. A friendship began right there. We all need a little help from angels sometimes. I had Renee in Orlando, now I had Adele. Get really sick and vulnerable and you can spot an angel at a hundred paces. You can almost see the wings and the halo. Adele was in a controlled panic and dashed away to pull the doctor out of his consultation, to see me at once.

Before leaving, she told me to finish up the last patch of wound cleaning myself. I was surprised by this and then she leaned into me and said with matronly authority: 'Jamie, you have to try and help yourself wherever and whenever you can. That's crucial to your recovery. We will look after you with everything we've got but you must, must look to help yourself. Try it and you'll soon see what I mean.' Not a day has gone by when those words haven't come back to me. She was saying: empower yourself, Jamie, break free of the humiliation of dependency. Ever since, I have not asked anyone to perform a task I might do myself, no matter what the effort. If I could do my own plastic surgery at home, I would.

In a few minutes, she was back with Dr Sudip Ghosh, the top burns consultant at Stoke Mandeville. He stood before my naked body, chin in his hand, biting down on his lower lip, shaking his head.

'When did Chelmsford discharge you?'

'Last night.'

'Well, you're our patient now. Sister Adele will arrange the preparation of your room. You are going to be with us for some time, I'm afraid. I'll come and see you when you are settled in.'

He left the room, Adele started rewrapping me with clean dressings and bandages and the tears stung the skin of my cheeks.

It would be 18 months before Stoke Mandeville discharged me.

19

> 'What manner of men are they that the wear the maroon beret? They are firstly all volunteers and are toughened by physical training. As a result they have infectious optimism and that offensive eagerness which comes from well-being ... They have the highest standards in all things ... They are, in fact, men apart – every man an emperor.'

So wrote Field Marshal Bernard Montgomery, 1st Viscount Montgomery of Alamein about the Parachute Regiment and it was to this elite military unit that, in 2003, I turned my focus at the end of my third and penultimate year at university, all other major OTC challenges exhausted for the time being. I knew all about the Paras. Who didn't? It was probably the one military outfit any man in a British street could name. The Royal Marines have unique qualities of their own but if Britain finds itself in a serious fight, it will be the Paras to whom they turn to act as the spearhead.

I had been reading up on them and I wanted a piece of their action, I wanted to accept their challenge – the fabled 'P' Company (Pegasus Company) selection course, which was open to all arms of the military, including the OTC. Outside Special Forces, 'P' Company is the hardest of all selection courses alongside the Royal Marines' Commando Training Programme. And some argue it's harder than Special Forces Selection because it lasts for three continuous, gruelling weeks. It is not broken down into parts. Besides, half the SAS were drawn from the Paras.

Back from Norway, the Cambridge University OTC quickly dominated my life once again, a little to the detriment of my academic studies, it must be admitted. I was just about on top of my studies, but I was under no illusions, from the marks I was getting for my course work, that I was heading for any better than an average-to-good grading in my finals. I didn't mind. As far as I was concerned, and so long as I didn't get a third, my achievements and experiences gained through the OTC, when added to my academic qualifications, were going to give me the notional equivalent of a first-class honours degree. If the idea of a university was for the graduate to emerge from it a better person, to build some character, to open up a range of life choices and career opportunities, then I was heading for a distinction.

I signed up for the pre-Parachute selection, meaning I wouldn't receive my 'wings' until I completed the jump element of the course at a later date. But jumping out of an aircraft was a one-off, a case of overcoming deep-seated fears. That held no terrors for me. But the main part of the course, held at Catterick Garrison in North Yorkshire, is a remorseless ordeal of pain. Completing a Cambrian Patrol was a triumph, a badge of honour for life, but from what I had heard, it was a challenge dwarfed in scale and intensity by 'P' Company – a course designed to push body, mind and soul to the limits of endurance day after day, week after week. If I passed the course and I made the jumps later on, there was nothing in theory to stop me joining the Paras.

But even if I was to make it through the three weeks – and most don't – what worried me the most was the thought that all that monumental effort could be for nothing, that I could blow it all in 60 seconds right at the end. Because, when those contestants still standing stagger in from the field for a final time, their very last kilojoule of energy seeping from their shattered bodies, they are obliged to enter the ring to prove their fighting spirit in the Paras' notorious 'milling' contest. I was strong, fit and determined but I was not a big lad, and I had never much gone in for pub or street fighting. Not since primary school, at least, when I learned for the first time that a lad should pick his fights wisely. I had come across some Paras and I could only hope I would be paired with someone roughly my build.

Officially, the Paras describe milling as 'controlled physical aggression' but anyone who has witnessed a milling bout will tell you that, in reality, it is just a savage fight that would probably end in serious injury if it went on for any longer than its wild 60 seconds. There is good reason why outsiders are strictly barred from attending. It's a Para thing. For their eyes only.

I was one of only two from Cambridge OTC to put themselves up for 'P' Company that year. The other was my mate Dan and we went into training as a pair in the dunes of the Norfolk coast, full packs on our backs. We stayed with Dan's gran in the traditional seaside town of Sheringham and we were feeling 'pretty butch' when we packed up our Bergens and got ready to set out for Catterick ... until we squeezed into Gran's tiny white Nissan Micra and whined our way up the A1. On arrival at the garrison, we endured a few chuckles from the men on the boom barrier at the guardhouse and we made sure to pull up out of sight and leave the 'granny-mobile' in the far corner of the car park.

We had every reason to be very nervous as we made our way to sign in and collect our kit. I had been warned about the drawbacks of being an officer in the making. NCOs like to work a young officer hard – and that's only partly because the army expects more from its leaders. Non-commissioned officers (NCOs), the Rodneys, love an opportunity to show the Ruperts who really runs the army. Of the 100 or so on the course, only about a dozen were officers or cadets. They were given white T-shirts, the NCO candidates red, with green for the privates and lance-corporals, or lance-jacks as they are known. I was handed a white T-shirt with the number 12 on the front. For the next three weeks that would be my name – 'White Twelve!' I never heard it spoken, only shouted. I had been warned to expect a little more attention from the instructors – and I sure got it.

The first two weeks were brutal. The instructors call it train-ing; the participants 'beasting'. I lost so much weight my buttocks disappeared. There was just skin, plus the ball head of my femur bones. But the real pain, the true challenge, was just about to begin: Test Week. It was fast and furious and agonising from the off, every day its own special nightmare, starting with a 10-miler over hill terrain in full kit with rifle, total weight of 50 pounds, to be completed in under 1 hour 50 minutes.

Next up the dreaded trainasium – a steel framework assault course, 55 feet above the ground. No great skill or stamina required – just a straight-up test of courage, haring along peril-ously narrow gangplanks and jumping into nets over huge yawning drops, punching an arm into the mesh, hoping it found a hole. The log race is considered one of the hardest events, an eight-man team heaving a telegraph pole for two miles over the hills. The two-mile march looked like respite on paper, but it is nothing but, carried out in full kit and to be run in under 18 minutes. Then there's the steeplechase, effectively a sprint over two miles and ending in a ground assault course. The stretcher race is a killer too, lugging a 175-pound dead weight for five miles. If you have made it that far, the week draws to an end with the 20-mile endurance march in full kit to be completed in under four hours and ten minutes.

Every event is point-scored, apart from the trainasium, which is a straight pass or fail. The course instructors look as if they walked straight out of a comic book of characters – all senior NCOs, each 15 stone-plus of solid muscle and complete with twitching handlebar tashes and thick sideburns. Face fashion hasn't moved on for the Para sergeant. But there is nothing amusing about these cartoon characters. These are the grizzled veterans of the Falklands, Northern Ireland and the Gulf Wars, the scariest men in the British Army. If there is late-night trouble on the garrison, the Regimental Sergeant Major sends in one of them to sort it out. The miscreant will take one punch and wake up in the infirmary. They are not a myth. They are a living, tash-bristling, musclebound reality and those under their command – and probably their officers too – go about in quaking fear of them.

The best part of the experience was the food and sleep. Without copious amounts of the former and a just sufficient amount of the latter, no one would ever pass. The human body, no matter how fit, and the spirit, no matter how resolute, have their limits. There are four huge meals a day, including a double-sized full English breakfast and as much porridge as you can get down, but that still wasn't enough fuel for the calorie furnaces our bodies had become. Every day, we dwindling band of participants jogged over to the on-site Tesco to load up on bananas, full-fat milk, energy bars and boxes of Snickers and Mars Bars.

From the very first, several contestants dropped out of the running every day and by the time Test Week came around, only 40 of the original 100 remained. The 20-miler at the end of the week was the closest I came to holding up my hands in surrender – or rather, dropping into the dirt. I started the course weighing 11 stone 5 pounds, but was down to 10 stone 4 after the first fortnight. I was now burning muscle, my fat stores cleared out, cramming in the Snicker bars as fast as I could chew them. At the 15-mile point, I was running on empty, about to go down, reeling like a slobbering drunk, but I made it, delirious and disorientated, and staggered over the finish line.

Many who have completed both courses say they found 'P' Company harder than Special Forces Selection. Both demand formidable powers of endurance, but they are different animals and any comparison between the two is a false one. The main difference is that on Selection, the candidate is on his own so he can pace himself, up to a point. If he's about to drop, he can take a quick breather, he won't be letting anyone down and he won't have a big moustache in his ear screaming and spitting fire and brimstone. In 'P' Company, the participants are watched every yard of the way. There is nowhere to hide. The scrutiny, the roaring of encouragement and abuse never flags. Everything is conducted at high speed, full tilt, best effort – often in teams and you can't let down the team. By several country miles, and then some, Test Week was the most punitive experience of my life.

And, just when I thought I could soak up no more punishment, it was time to go milling.

Milling is similar to boxing in that the contestant wears gloves, head protection and a mouth guard, it takes place in a ring of sorts before a baying crowd, and the aim is to overwhelm your opponent with fists while blocking and dodging the incoming blows. Officially, there is no winner and no loser. Skill doesn't come into the reckoning. It's all about aggression. It's about the fight in the man, how he might react behind enemy lines, unarmed and cornered. It is a Para ritual and anyone who has competed never forgets it. If Sky Sports broadcast it, it would be a box-office smash. Terrifying to watch, it is manifoldly more so to contest.

It takes place in the old, echoing gymnasium on the base. If you thought the rest was tough, the milling is 'nails', I kept being told before heading north. When we filed in, it was as if we had walked into a nineteenth-century public school initiation ceremony.

Two rows of low gym benches on each side formed a square, the action to take place within it. Behind the benches, on all sides, more Paras formed ranks to watch the gladiatorial spectacle. On the far side, a six-foot-high stack of gym mats and on top of them, three chairs: the Officer Commanding in the centre, like the Emperor, flanked by the RSM and a senior sergeant, Mexican-style handlebar moustaches down to their jawbones, clipboards in their giant fists. If I wasn't nervous before, I was now. I had an audience of hard-nuts to humiliate myself before.

We all formed up and a sergeant walked up and down, detailing us into groups based roughly on height and weight. A group of monsters on one side, and the Liquorice Allsorts on the other, the stocky, the lanky and the wiry. Then we were paired off for our bouts.

I took one look at my opponent and smiled inwardly: young lad, barely out of school, green shirt, same height and build. I am no fighter, but I can handle myself if needs must. I'm tidy. I'd been a copper. I was confident I could have him. But the adrenaline was flooding my system, the 'fight–flight' reflex triggering a cascade of the stuff. The prospect of performing on a stage before a raucous, bloodthirsty mob cranked up the emotions still higher.

Ours was the second fight so I now knew what to expect. 'White 12! Green 9!' the RSM hollered and we stepped through the ranks and into the 'ring' up to the ref, the room utterly silent again. We stood toe to toe, nose to nose, forehead to forehead.

The ref leaned in and said: 'You got sixty seconds, it's best effort. Standby ... and mill!' I exploded, the lad in green exploded, the room exploded. It was an explosion of adrenaline, an explosion of noise, an explosion of flailing fists. It wasn't a life-and-death struggle. I could have just walked out and said, *Fuck this for a game of soldiers*, and gone back to uni and the OTC, the abuse from the room ringing in my ears: *Go on, grab your rail grant and fuck off back to Toytown*. No true shame in that and to hell with what they thought. But I'd be damned if I was going to half kill myself over three weeks, only to screw it all up in the very last minute for want of courage. So, right then, it sure felt like life-or-death.

Every contestant went for it because they knew that, if they'd been weak on one of the earlier runs or exercises, they could maybe win it back, get over the line, with a display of raw aggression and animal spirit. In the court of warrior opinion, everyone in the room, not just the judges on high, needed no more than 60 seconds to see if a guy had the character to be a Para.

I had no idea how I was doing on the course point scoring. Nor did my adversary and the two of us piled into each other like we would keep going until one of us stopped breathing. Short of kicking and biting, it was no holds barred. The ref stopped the fight after about 45 seconds to check the guy in green. His eyes were puffing, his lip was up and blood ran from his nose. My features weren't much prettier.

'You all right, kid?'

'Yes, staff!' he shouted, and we hurled ourselves at each other again, me getting the better of him once again. At the bell, I was in no doubt that I had prevailed. I'd put on a brilliant show of violence. The smile pushing at my mouth disappeared when the Officer Commanding boomed my judgement.

To the kid in green: 'Top effort, lad, you really dug in there, showed some guts.'

To me: 'White 12, I'm not bloody happy with that. Your heart wasn't in it. I'm putting you in again.'

What the fuck? My heart sunk but I got what was going on, the psychology behind the ruling. I stood on the sidelines, watching another 20 bouts, 20 minutes of ferocious battering, blood and sweat spraying the floor, wild cheers and shouts rolling around the hall. You can do a lot of damage to a body in 60 seconds and a couple needed immediate medical attention on the sidelines. The officers had it toughest of all – for the NCOs and ranks this was their only chance to batter one legally. I eyed up the gorillas, wondering which one I'd get.

My second bout was the last of the day and I had identified my opponent by then – the guy who won his first bout easy and got the same dressing-down from the OC as I had. I had got to know him a little over the previous few weeks. He was a serving Royal Marine, a lance-corporal, a little older, a little taller but much heavier, bent nose, plastered in tats, Welsh. He was doing 'P' Company for the hell of it, see how it compared to the Commando course. He had nothing to prove to anyone. He just liked the pain, the effort, the sense of triumph.

There was total silence in the room as we squared up, the ref with his hands on our shoulders, me leaning back on my heels to take a quick step away. I knew what the gorilla was thinking: *I am going to eat this little whippet. There's nothing of him. And he's a fucking cadet.*

' … and mill!'

The room erupted in a roar. 'Fucking have him! … Do the fucker! … Get in! … Knock him out! … Do him!'

The Paras weren't rooting for either of us, they just wanted the violence, the primal thrill of a fight to the death, or as close you could get to one within the law. If anyone, it was probably me they wanted to prevail, the little underdog against the Royal Marine. There has never been love lost between Marines and Paras.

It was a cartoon blur of windmilling arms, but the Marine was getting the better of it. A good three stone heavier, he used his superior weight advantage and longer reach to gain the upper hand. I felt the blood sluicing from my nose and mouth, one of my eyes starting to close. The ref yanked us apart, gave me the count. I tried not to sway. We'd barely been going 20 seconds at each other. It was difficult to tell if the fog in my head was the adrenaline of the moment, or the pummelling I was taking.

'You fit to go on? You want to go on?'

'Yes, staff!'

And I did. I really did want to go on. Something was coming over me. Call it what you want – an indomitable will to win, survival instinct, divine inspiration, an extra pint of adrenaline in the blood, whatever. My brain was telling me that if I didn't step up, make a superhuman effort, this Welsh ape was going to cause me serious damage. It was the only time in my life I had experienced this feeling of invincibility, a need to win at all costs, push myself way, way beyond what I understood to be the limits of my strength.

An observer would say that I snapped, that I had become possessed by a demonic force. My eyes were bulging, and my body tensed as though I was having a seizure. I put my head down and I piled into the astonished Marine, the Paras bellowing themselves hoarse. Never again would I ever experience this surge of extreme power. It was almost supernatural. I was taking punches too, but I was going full tilt and the balance of power switched. Time appeared to slow down. I was punching in slow motion. The uproar became a muffled din. No one had been expecting this fightback, the racing snake against the king of the primates.

I drove him foot by foot into the corner in a barrage of punches to the head, face and body. One to the ribcage made the Marine drop his elbow to protect it and I unleashed a welter of punches to his unprotected face. I had him over the second bench, the Paras scattering, when the bell rang out and the ref pulled me off the prostrate Welshman.

The ref led us back to the centre of the ring, our faces streaming blood, the Marine clutching his rib, and the OC said, 'Good scrap, lads, strong finish, White 12. Now everyone go get yourselves cleaned up.'

And that was it. We all filed out as if nothing had happened. The Marine and I slapped each other on the back, both trembling a little, lungs heaving, sweat and blood gushing.

'Well done, mate.'

'And you, pal.'

We jogged away for a quick shower, and then out to the parade ground to find out if we had passed or failed the three weeks. The 'P' Company survivors creaked and groaned around the barracks, shattered, bloodied and bruised. I towelled myself down, the anxiety mounting in my aching limbs, slowly pulled on some clean fatigues, a fresh white T-shirt, and shaped the OTC beret on my head. At noon, we were all in formation, standing at ease. There was no ceremony, no speeches, no congratulations. The Officer Commanding just called out a name and number, the guy stood to attention and judgement was delivered, a terse 'Pass' or 'Fail'.

'Johnson, Green 9 – fail … Hunter, Red 22 – pass …'

He spoke as if he was reading out a shopping list, absolutely no emotion one way or the other. Just the plain facts, flatly delivered. A surprising number were being failed, about a quarter of them. My nose still leaking blood, I was one of the last, and by the time it came I was convinced I was going to hear the dreaded 'F' word.

'Hull, White 12 …'

I stood to.

'Pass!'

The tension dropped from my shoulders and I had to bite my lip so as not to yelp with joy – or, relief, more accurately.

Again, that was it. The group dispersed, gathered their Bergens, got into their cars or trains and went back whither they'd come, pass or fail.

My mate Dan had passed too, but our exhaustion trumped our elation and we drove back down the A1 saying nothing, letting the radio wash over us. It wasn't until we pulled over for fuel that we formally recognised one another's achievement, giving each other a hug and a slap on the back. We didn't need to say anything.

Dan went on to join the Paras, following in the footsteps of his father. I was eligible too. I just needed to do complete the jump element, get my wings. I had done the hardest part. There was nothing to stop me driving straight to 4 Para HQ in London and signing up for the territorial unit of the famous regiment.

But that decision could wait. I was suffering concussion from the milling. My head hurt for days, but not as much as my body, and it was a week before I felt fully recovered from the assault to which I had subjected myself. But I didn't care. I was glowing on the inside. I had long ago discovered that I had been blessed with some gifts of willpower, the grit to keep going when most throw in the towel. But 'P' Company had revealed new depths of character of which I had no suspicion. It turned out I was a fighter after all. I never knew that.

20

The insurance people couldn't move me on fast enough from Orlando, then Chelmsford couldn't wait to see the raw, mouldy back of me. I was the toxic bomb in a game of pass-the-parcel. I understand why, but it still hurt. Maybe I wasn't used to being vulnerable and dependent, maybe I'd get used to it. I have no idea whether Chelmsford pulled a fast one, knowing full well that Stoke Mandeville would have to take me in. I have no idea either whether Chelmsford tried to have me transferred but someone at Stoke Mandeville, knowing I was a walking sponge of invasive infections, politely turned down the request.

I wanted to be in Stoke Mandeville and I wanted the hell out of Chelmsford for sure. But not like that. I wanted to be transferred, not chucked out. Dress it up as you like, but that's what I was – I was chucked out on to the street. Not even a non-emergency ambulance to take me home. I was transported in a private car to a camp bed in a cramped living room with no medical facilities. I was made to work it out for myself, the caution over my condition tossed to a strong, cold wind. If I had tried to push on and continue with my recovery at home, not gripe about it, it's unsettling to think what might have happened.

I don't moan easy but within a day of leaving Chelmsford I was effectively imploring for admission to a new hospital and I believe that merits a good whinge. If Stoke Mandeville had turned me away, agreeing with Chelmsford's appraisal of my condition, I would have sat there begging like a man on death row for a reprieve. Luckily, Adele and Dr Ghosh needed only one look at me. I didn't even need to be examined. The fact I was still an in-patient in Stoke Mandeville 18 months after the morning I walked in for the first time is its own evidence that my discharge from Chelmsford was exactly 18 months premature.

· · ·

I ended up being one of the longest-serving burn patients Stoke Mandeville had ever had. It was a happier experience than Chelmsford, but proper happiness was a red herring, not even on the menu. My happiness levels were at zero. The quality of care, the quality of the hospital, the comfort of my room – all the external, material factors that add up to some sort of contentment in ordinary life, were irrelevant to my feelings about myself, my place in the world.

I have occasionally wondered whether I would have felt even the smallest stirrings of happiness had I remained and regained consciousness in the state-of-the-art, superbly resourced Orlando Regional Medical Center. I doubt it. You look the same in a mirror wherever you are holding it. A corridor to shuffle down is the same on both sides of the Atlantic.

As at Chelmsford, I had a love–hate relationship with a few of the nurses at Stoke Mandeville. They worked very hard for me, but I was cranky and sullen much of the time, downright rude even. Clinical staff can be charming and kind as saints, the room bright and fresh, the meals cordon bleu, you can be fed a stream of the best films, handed the best books ever written, they could give you a blowjob to help you off to sleep – but you're still lying in a hospital suffering pain and frustration and not getting on with your life.

My active life is no more important than the next man's, but I suffered my injuries when I was at the very peak of my physical capabilities. I was in that bracket of age and experience when Premier League footballers get transferred for tens of millions. I was like a thoroughbred horse in the stalls thrashing about for the gates to open. It's the reason why I decided to use the free month before deployment to acquire my pilot's licence. I needed to fill every day constructively, to feel purposeful, that I was getting the max out of life. I had an urgency to be active, bordering on hyperactivity and, no kidding, I believe this impulse was almost a certifiable mental health condition. For 15 years, I just could not sit still. I had to be doing something all the time. I wasn't happy unless I was sweating, my lungs were burning or I was framing another certificate for my wall. Pinning me to a bed for however many months and years was just about the best way to drive me insane. A bookworm could probably handle it, but then again, the meds make you so hazy, concentration is hard and reading is not easy. You're sedentary, sure, but reading is an activity. You have to focus. I existed in a dull haze of pain and boredom.

It had reached the point when going for a skin graft became an event I looked forward to, in spite of the searing pain I knew I was going to feel as soon as I came around after the procedure. At least it was an event, it was progress and having a stranger run a carpentry plane over my raw skin beats staring at an off-white ceiling listening to Steve Wright every time for me.

These were big grafts they were carrying out now that I was a bit stronger. My arse cheeks, inner thighs and areas of my back offered the best skin. The dermatome, the instrument they use to peel off a roll of skin, really is similar to the plane used in wood-work. It is run over the harvest area, as the plane is over a length of wood, and the skin curls up into a roll just like a wood shaving. The roll of skin is then applied to a piece of sticky resin to hold it flat before it is meshed by a special machine, stretching it so you get more bang for your buck. When it's ready to be grafted it looks like a string vest with diamond-shaped holes, a patch of living gauze, perforated to allow blood and serum to leak from the wound. The idea is that the treated site can breathe, and the cells below get to work on growing it into the finished article. Once you are no longer unsettled by the process, the surgeon will tell you this part of the process is less like carpentry and more like leatherwork.

You want your own skin because it is the most likely to take, but that means stripping away one area of skin to cover another – robbing Peter to pay Paul, as one of the surgeons put it. The donor site being smaller than the wound site, you are therefore always taking one step back to take two forward or, occasionally when the skin doesn't take, just the step back. I'd like to say that you get used to skin grafts, but you don't. You are under general anaesthetic, of course, but when you come around, the pain is intense, similar to severe burns, in fact. But there was a certain satisfaction in seeing the quilt being stitched together and the drama of the event added some colour to an otherwise grey existence.

Just as grafting skin from your own body is a necessary evil, taking that hit for Team Body, so too with the meds. From the day of my accident, I had been on high-dose, high-strength antibiotics and painkillers, together with a cabinet load of others for local, less dramatic problems, like ointments for my eyes and ears. My hearing, in my right ear especially, had been impaired by the force of the explosion and I suffered from tinnitus, a constant fizzing and whirring in my head. My eyesight was a little blurred from the burn scarring and the ophthalmologist became another regular specialist in my life. The pills, liquids and creams could be measured in buckets and barrels and dispensed as wholesale goods. I had also absorbed huge quantities of sedative for the induced coma and immeasurable amounts of general anaesthetic for my operations and procedures. I would have died very early on without the antibios, and I would not have stopped screaming and wailing without the analgesics, the sedatives and palliatives, the tanks of Entonox gas. They were essential but inevitably they made me feel down, feeding my gloom, and it's not natural for a body to be coursing with so many alien substances.

I was in one of the six rooms on Ward 11 of the Burns Unit. I had it to myself and it was a good-quality room. There was a modern television on the wall, a window from which I could see some sky and a comfortable armchair for my visitors. No flowers or plants were allowed for fear of infection. It was a lifeless, sterile, spotlessly clean environment. It was sepsis or dahlias and I was happy to pass on the dahlias.

The rooms came off the hub of the nurses' station like spokes of a wheel, but unlike Orlando, there was no glass door so I could only hear what was going on in the rest of the ward. Doctors and nurses don't shout so, when I was on my own, the only human voices I heard from the beyond were the other patients scream-ing in agony or groaning and sobbing in the night. No one is admitted to a bed in a burns unit if they're feeling comfortable. Chemical burns, electrical burns, scalding liquid burns, fireworks, barbeques, house fires, car fires ... Stoke Mandeville had them all during my stay.

It's very hard to feel other people's pain. We are programmed to forget our own episodes in order that we will not be fright-ened to take the risks and suffer a repeat of the agony thereafter. A mother having a second child is the best example of that phenomenon. It is only when you are in the same degree of pain as another that you can empathise with them at a meaningful level and my heart went out to my fellow sufferers on Ward 11 every time they cried out.

I had dozens of visitors at Chelmsford and Stoke Mandeville, but the flood soon became a trickle. Most came only once and I was grateful for the effort, but there was never much to talk about, no common ground, and that can start to weigh heavily on the atmosphere quite quickly. I didn't want to hear about their relatively happy and pain-free existence, them getting on with life, and there wasn't a great deal to report from my end. What to say? *I had a very acceptable chicken Diane yesterday. Mashed potato was a little cold, but the peas were done just right. I think it's shepherd's pie tonight ... I had fun watching the square of grey sky through my window this afternoon ...*

Mostly my visitors were family and old mates from the army, university and Leighton Buzzard, but it's funny who turns up. I could barely remember the names of a few of them. They tended to be the ones I had been at junior school with and, 20 years on, some were as unrecognisable as me and hard to place. Word had got around about my accident, and there was a handful of visits that made me wonder whether I was just a curiosity, a one-man freak show with free entry. There were half-a-dozen people I genuinely did not know, in tow with people I knew just a little. I couldn't help but feel they had just come for the thrill of a gawp at my hideously disfigured face, like rubberneckers at a motorway wipeout.

A few friends came or got in touch many times, and not necessarily the ones you'd expect. To them, I owe an eternal debt of gratitude. Chief among that number was my old OTC mate Pete Mash, a brilliant Cambridge scientist, but more of him later. He plays a big part in my new life. The person whose kindness touched me the most, back in the UK, was a guy I grew up with but hadn't seen for years.

Matthew Hawkes had come to see me a few times in Chelmsford. That was a long schlep for him, driving down from Hemel

Hempstead. Commuting to London every day, he did quite enough travelling as it was. When I was admitted to Stoke Mandeville, he came to see me every week. He was the model visitor and exemplary friend. He didn't do chirp. He rarely told me about what was going on his life and rarely probed me with questions about how I was 'feeling', having worked out that the answer was self-explanatory. He just sat there and often not a great deal would be said. I felt comfortable in his presence – maybe it's true about the deep bonds of friendship forged in childhood – and after a time, at my lowest moments, I unloaded on him.

There was a great deal of rage, grief and fear in me, and I had been trying to be a man about it, tough it out, process it all myself. I had refused the offer of psychotherapy support believing I had the strength to cope, but there was also an element of not wanting to unload and share with a stranger. But with Matt, I felt no embarrassment, no compulsion to play it tough, and from time to time I cried without restraint. He never tried to talk me up in those moments. He just sat in the armchair, his presence the only reassurance I needed. Finally, when I was done dumping on him and feeling in a better place, he'd get up to go and tell me he'd see me next week. No chirp, no chat-show tears.

I was having to get used to this crying business. Before my accident, I could count on one hand the occasions I got tearful. When Mum and Dad split was one. Another was getting a rollicking from Mum when I was about seven after I downed a bottle of banana-flavoured medicine and had to have my stomach pumped. I am told crying is good for us and I am sure that's true. Trouble is, it doesn't look or feel so great if you're in the SAS. I'm meant to be tough, to have that extra level of resilience to see out extreme physical and mental pressure. That's true, but Special Forces operatives bleed, burn and shed tears too. If the designers of an Special Forces course made candidates suffer 65 per cent three-degree burns and not cry as a prerequisite for selection, you would end up with an extremely small and elite unit.

I cried a lot in Chelmsford and Stoke Mandeville, and I don't care who knows it. It was rarely the physical pain – and I am not just saying that to sound butch. It was the emotional pain. My morale crumbled and then collapsed. It was the mirror that triggered the implosion. As soon as I could walk a little, I was seeing myself everywhere in reflections not just when I hobbled to the bathroom. When I snapped off *The Jeremy Kyle Show*, there I was staring back at myself in the blackened television screen. When I practised walking down the corridor, the windows became a gallery of my own horror show. Even if the reflection was faint, the distortion of my features was so great it jumped out at me.

I looked monstrous, but my aesthetic appearance was only a small cause of my despair. It was my face as a symbol for what my life had become and held out for me. It was the finger on a trigger for the self-loading, semi-automatic of my incontinent grief. What girl was going to hold hands with that in a cinema or down the High Street? Who'd want to marry that? What kids would want jump to sit on that knee? What employer would send that out to bat for the company? I hated the sight of myself and increasingly I hated the very thought of myself. If you don't like yourself, there is no joy, there is no hope, there is no life for you out there. The only joy in my life was the occasional and mild relief from intense pain that came from a hit of morphine, the satisfaction of hunger from the eating of a meal, the quenching of thirst with a glass of water. Some visitors said, 'Well, at least you've got a TV.' But I hated the TV, and it wasn't just the constant sound of chirp. It was because the television was a reminder of what I could no longer do: run around a track, kiss a girl, fight in a war, lie on a beach, climb a mountain. I can't even say I was pleased to see my mother because I knew that her life was sinking in step with mine. What a burden I was for a mother! No loving son wants to be a burden to his mother.

I was better off dead. So that's what I decided to do. To die. I had a laptop I could operate with a finger on my left hand – my right arm was still healing Hitler – and one evening, after a prolonged bout of tears, I launched my correspondence with Dignitas. When I pressed Send and my email winged its way across the Alps to their HQ in Switzerland, it was the first time I had felt happy in over a year. I smiled, swallowed my meds and fell into a sleep undisturbed by nightmares.

21

I had turned 28 during the 'P' Company course earlier in the summer of 2003 and I wanted to get on with life. My appetite for achieving personal goals had become insatiable. Studying was fine, learning languages great, a degree was valuable, playing sport and going to the pub were fun – but it was nowhere near enough to fulfil my raging energy.

I didn't know for sure if I wanted to pursue a career in the Armed Forces, but I certainly wanted the option. All I had to do was jump out of an aircraft a few times and I'd be a Paratrooper. But, after OTC and 'P' Company, I was going to be in the happy position of being able to put myself forward for any regiment I liked and be confident of admission.

I was spoiled for choice beyond the military too. I could re-join the police, become a diving instructor, mountain leader, ski instructor, adventure tourism guide or, like most of my fellow graduates, armed with my degree and all my extra-curricular achievements, I could head into London and qualify as some sort of professional and make some money. It was unlikely that my itchy feet would allow me to settle for a desk-jockey career at this stage, but it was reassuring to know the option was there.

The full course at Sandhurst lasts the better part of a year but there are shorter courses for those who have passed many of the basics as cadets or reservists – or if the candidates are non-combat professionals whose skills are highly prized in the military, medics in the main. I needed only to pass the shortest, four-week course. That began in August and rolled into September, overlapping with the beginning of my fourth and final year at university.

When I asked the Dean of Faculties for a special dispensation to arrive for term two weeks late, my request was declined. So, I went anyway. No one would ever know. I'd say I'd been sick and then get my head down to catch up on the lectures and essays I had missed. My degree involved only seven hours contact time a week. Besides, the lazier students never turned up to lectures or tutorials anyhow, mainly because they were hungover, stoned over or simply couldn't be arsed to get out of bed. I thought that becoming a commissioned officer in Her Majesty's Armed Forces was a good enough excuse to skip a fortnight of half-hearted study – especially when both the weekends would be spent at the OTC anyhow.

It was a baking hot day in August 2003 when I stepped off the train at Camberley, a 30-mile hop from London and, the nerves nibbling at my guts, made my way through the pedestrianised shopping precinct and north into the leafy residential streets of the nondescript Surrey dormitory town.

The Royal Military Academy Sandhurst (RMAS) is one of the most eminent military colleges in the world. If not the most. Founded as the Royal Military College in 1801 to improve the leadership quality and field skills of the officer class, it has been doing exactly that ever since. Before then, unlike the Royal Navy and later the Royal Air Force, if you were sufficiently wealthy or well-connected, you could just buy your commission in the British Army, take immediate command of hundreds, even thousands of soldiers and head straight into battle. A lad from the back streets of Leighton Buzzard need not have applied.

Britain's navy, the enforcer of empire, was a formidable power back then, its strength shown in defeating the combined fleets of mighty France and Spain at Trafalgar in 1805. But the army, rarely called upon and few in number, was a very poor relation. Sandhurst put that right. Ever since, it has produced officers of a standard as high as anywhere in the world. Such is its prowess that armies from many countries send their own cadets to be trained from scratch, or to be polished to a higher standard. Heads of state, top-ranking generals and captains of industry have all passed through the Corinthian pillars of Sandhurst's Old College.

After 'P' Company, I might have been forgiven for imagining that Sandhurst was going to be a bit of a posh picnic by comparison. But I'd had enough experience of military life and heard all the stories about Sandhurst to know what lay in store. No one breezes in and out of Sandhurst and the designers of the consolidated course had packed a heavy and exacting schedule.

So, giving my jacket and tie a rare outing, the nerves now gnawing at my guts, I presented myself at the unobtrusive stone guardhouse and made my way into the inner sanctum of the British Army.

It wasn't my fitness or my weapon-handling skills that were going to come under scrutiny. It was my character. Sandhurst is about leadership, making sure you have the requisite personality traits to guide and inspire those under your command. Traditionally, a great number of the Sandhurst intake come from private schools and arrive with oven-ready self-confidence (sometimes a little too much of it, and knocking some of that out is the instructors' order of the day).

These days, for most making their way through those gates, Sandhurst is their opportunity to start acquiring that self-belief. Fitness is only one element, a prerequisite almost. It is one thing to run yourself into the ground over the Welsh mountains or Yorkshire Dales, taking spittle-coated orders from scary NCOs.

It is quite another to learn the craft of leadership, reverse that relationship and grow the balls to issue the orders to – and earn the respect of – those self-same NCOs, the backbone of the British Army.

To walk through those gates, out of suburbia and into the grounds of the military academy, is to pass into another dimension, a world quite apart from the everyday sights and experiences outside. A new world, a new life. The setting is dominated by the Regency-era Old College, its pillared cream-white facade overlooking the parade ground and aprons of immaculately manicured lawns. Beyond it lies almost 700 acres of parkland, sports fields, lakes and training area. Sandhurst looks like a very grand old school – and that's pretty well what it is. But there's only one course on offer: leadership.

I stood taking it all in, memories of my errant youth pressing into the front of my mind, not quite believing that I, Jamie Hull – ex-scally, petty criminal and rebel without applause – was four weeks away from becoming a commissioned officer in Her Majesty's Armed Forces. Who'd have thought? Certainly not my teachers, my parents, my mates or the local bobbies – and least of all myself. I pictured myself, the wiry tearaway down by the railway tracks in Leighton Buzzard skinning a joint and slugging at a bottle of Strongbow, weighing up which High Street shop to rob that day. And now this – Sandhurst! It's only 50 miles from Leighton to Sandhurst, but for me the journey had been an epic odyssey.

I was already a trained soldier. You could throw me a gun and point me in the direction of battle and I'd know how to handle my weapon and handle myself. As I was soon to discover, that experience wasn't going to confer the advantages I might have expected. I had passed 'P' Company – and that made me a marked man. The training captain had read my profile and lined me up in his sights before I even stepped past the stone gatehouse. It was a compliment of sorts, but it sure wouldn't feel like it.

A regime more removed from the leisurely life of university is hard to imagine. The university student tends to rise when most people are either at work or on their way. The day might be made up of a lecture in the morning, a bit of study in the library if the mood takes in the afternoon, the odd coffee, maybe a bit of sport, and then off to the pub or Union for a couple of pints and home for a movie and maybe a joint and some casual sex. That's great. University is more than just devouring academic matter, passing exams and collecting a fancy certificate. It's a transitional period in life, a bridge between school and childhood on one side, and adulthood and the big wide world on the other. It is an enviable privilege to experience it.

At Sandhurst, the daily regime is the diametric opposite.

The day begins at five-thirty with a colour sergeant barking at you to jump to, get your hands off cocks and on to socks, get your lazy fucking arse out of bed ... Cadets sleep in cell-like rooms off a long corridor and each must keep his personal belongings, bed and open locker to the highest standards of order and cleanliness. The bed must be made so there is no hint of a crease, the clothes stacked on it no larger than a sheet of A4, all shirts facing the same way on the coat rail, and each item of the wash kit – toothbrush, paste, shampoo and deodorant – lined up on the shelf at an equal distance from the next, like soldiers on parade. At Sandhurst, they never tire of telling you that the road to glory starts with a perfectly folded sock.

Inspections are constant. There are inspections of kit, of your living space, your weapons, your boots, your Bergen – every possible area of you, and the way you present yourself and go about your daily business. The colour sergeant doesn't follow you into the toilet cubicle to assess your arse-wiping skills, but after a while you have the feeling that he might just do that. Cadets soon get the message (very) loud and (very) clear that the way we spend our days is the way we spend our lives. You carry out a task over and over until the activity becomes so routine it's second nature, you don't even know you're doing it, so that one day, out in the field, you are free to focus on what really matters.

The way I brought in the plane while it was on fire, going through every stage of the emergency protocol, may have owed something to what I had learned at Sandhurst about the importance of procedure. It's boring but crucial: repetition and practice are the foundations of good soldiering, perhaps the foundations of any good life. It might even save your life one day.

It was the same with the drill exercises we were made to practise on the parade ground. Boring as hell, up and down, up and down, left right, left right, but after a time, when we start on fieldcraft, we soon understood the point of the mindless square-bashing. The mindlessness is an essential part of it: doing something until it is automatic. But on exercises in the field, we learned that drill teaches you more than that. It teaches you about teamwork, about the individual making a contribution to the whole body of men. If one guy is out of step, they all look bad. Same goes out in the field when it really matters – one guy trips on his untied boot laces and breaks his leg, or his unclean weapon jams, then that person puts the whole unit in jeopardy.

The only element of the course that didn't tax me too hard was the fitness programme – the runs and assault courses. On the day I arrived, it was hardly possible for a human body to be in better condition. I'd whisper it quietly, but I actually quite liked being 'beasted', pushed to the limit of my endurance. I was the most self-competitive person I had ever met.

'Long days and short weeks' is how they describe the Sand-hurst experience and for me, by some distance, the hardest challenges were out in the field where we had to plan and carry out mock battlefield exercises. It was here that I became the moving target for the training captain and the NCOs who had marked my card before the course had even begun.

It was the toughest part of the course for us all because it was in fieldcraft and leadership roles that the instructors can really tell who's got it and who hasn't. And they make sure there's plenty of opportunities for you to screw up.

Leading up to the first platoon exercise, I had sensed I was attracting the attention of the hard-nosed training captain a little more than the others. As we milled around, waiting for instruction, the captain ran his eyes over the group and stopped when he got to me. I had been 'dicked'.

'Officer Cadet Hull, you will lead the attack on the enemy position.'

Knowing that honour was probably coming my way didn't lessen the anxiety that washed over me.

I was given a set of basic orders and a bit of time to prepare the assault. Awaiting us in the enemy positions were real infantry drafted in for the day to roleplay. Everyone is issued with blanks for their SA80 assault rifles in order to make the experience as realistic as possible. I thought I had devised a cunning plan to defeat my foe, opting for a frontal assault. My assumption was that the enemy would expect me to get clever and attack from the flanks, stretching their line and drawing their fire in two directions. I was going to double bluff the idiots.

As they moved up, the message runners kept bringing me fresh intelligence about the enemy's movement (fed by the training captain), forcing me to think fast on my feet and adapt my plan accordingly. The rush of information soon addled my judgement and I ceased to think clearly under the pressure, failing to make full use of my three sections.

In short, I screwed up. And Christ, did the training captain let me know it. The assault was called off halfway through, we mustered back at the forming-up point and the training captain let rip, 'tearing me a new arsehole', as they like to say.

My face just an inch away, the captain screamed, swore and sprayed me in spittle, the 30 other guys looking on nervously. The exercise was binned and we were marched back to the college in silence. It was the most humiliating moment of my life since the day my parents had come to take me home from the Milton Keynes police station. I stood and took the bollocking without flinching, but inside I was cut up, my confidence shot. After the Cambrians and 'P' Company, I'd come to regard myself as a good operator in the field. I'd never let myself down, I'd never let my comrades down. That belief lay in pieces as I went back to the dormitory and hurled my kit at my locker. Maybe the training captain was right? Maybe I wasn't as good as I thought?

What I didn't know was that a) there was a theatrical element in the captain's performance. It wasn't staged, but the instructors were going to make sure I screwed up whichever way I planned and led the assault. There was no way they were going to let me succeed, give me a pat on the back and we all happily trot back for a steaming shower and a nice hot supper. And b) they had probably chosen me because, with all my experience, I had shown I had some soldiering talent and an appetite for leadership and they wanted to push me really hard to see how I'd respond. They knew I could take the withering criticism. I did make a hash of it, but I was also being used as the crash-test dummy so that the others got the message.

Ask the instructors and commanders, and they will tell you they actually like to see failure at Sandhurst. It is almost encouraged. They want the cadets to experience it. The thinking is that it's only through failure that we learn. Sandhurst is all about self-development and part of that is to know your strengths, sure, but better still, to recognise your weaknesses. Honesty is prized – admit your fault, even to the men under your command and they will respect you more. Cover it up and they won't. They want you to think your way out of failure. No panic, take a knee, have a good think. I felt and said all the right things. I apologised to the captain, apologised to my men, admitted I had come up short and would do my best to learn from my failure. What I didn't do was argue my case, or show my despair – and that, at Sandhurst, counts as success.

The humiliation that shook me achieved the positive effect intended – for me and all the other cadets who were witness to it. I took the hit, but its reverberations were felt by all. I stepped up over the next couple of weeks, acknowledging to myself that I wasn't just there to add the last few coats of polish to the training I had been receiving at the OTC. One area in which I had palpably failed was in teamwork – I hadn't consulted enough with my comrades in the planning of the attack. To lead, I now understood, does not mean you avoid or shun the opinions of those around you. You listen, then you decide and issue orders. It's not just about telling others what to do.

In the exercises that followed, other cadets were singled out to lead and, as the course reached its conclusion, confidence rose across the entire intake – my shame having worked its magically galvanising effect. The final exercise arrived: the big one. It takes place over two days and two nights and it might just determine whether you are one of the deserving 80 per cent – roughly – who pass Sandhurst or one of the also-rans obliged to walk out the gates and start researching a new career.

I didn't have a thousand pounds in those days, but if I had, I would have bet the whole lot that the training captain was going to tell me to lead the all-important assault. This time it was against a company of Gurkhas, one of Britain's finest regiments. I almost stepped out from the group before the captain had opened his mouth. And guess what?

'Officer Cadet Hull, we haven't had the chance to see you lead since your appalling effort a couple of weeks ago. Let's hope you've had time to reflect on your abject failings. You will be in command at the start. Let's see how you get on this time.'

On this occasion, it was a major, the commanding officer of that course's intake, who made the announcement, my hard-nose training captain standing stony-faced at his side.

The platoon marched out under darkness and for the first 24 hours we performed regular manoeuvres, nothing too taxing. The leadership role was switched a couple of times and then, just as we were about to climb into their sleeping bags, a runner arrived from 'HQ' with a warning order, notifying the platoon we must conduct an attack at first light.

Any one of the 30 might have been chosen, and we were all a little skittish with nerves, bantering about who was going to draw the short straw. I knew full well who it was going to be and, sure enough, the rest of the platoon let out a sigh of relief that was almost a shout when the orders envelope was opened. It was an honour, but it felt like a shit-pie in the face.

Planning the attack, based on the intelligence provided, was the most important element. For a poor plan to lead to a successful attack, the enemy has to be even more incompetent – and that wasn't going to happen against the Gurkhas or any unit of the Regular Army, especially as they enjoyed superiority in numbers and ground position. It was only a mock-up but the stakes were so high, the air so tense, that I really did feel as if men might die if I screwed up. Forget 'P' Company, this was the hardest and most important test of my army experiences to date. If I was failed, then 'P' Company would mean nothing. I'd have to join the army as a private and work my way up from the bottom and that was something for which I did not have the patience. It could take 20 years to become an officer. I wanted to get on in the world.

The platoon sections were spread out over the terrain facing the enemy position. While they got their heads down, I worked through the night with my section commanders to devise a plan based on the initial briefing. Just when we felt happy with our tactics, fresh intelligence from 'HQ' would arrive and we would have to alter the plan in the light of it. We did as we had been taught, building a model to scale of the enemy positions, using any materials to hand – twigs, coins, matchboxes – adjusting it with every fresh bulletin throughout the small hours.

It was gone four in the morning when we destroyed the model. I briefed the section commanders with their separate tasks and then summoned all the men for the Order Group. The 'O' Group is the meeting in which a commander spells out the plan of attack or manoeuvre, ordinarily just to the key personnel in the unit but, in this case, to everyone on the exercise. It was a good plan, but I knew it wouldn't survive the first impact with the enemy. We had met the Gurkhas before the exercise. Their reputation as superb soldiers has been well earned over their 200-year service with the British Army. They were fantastic guys too. I loved meeting them, but I knew those big toothy grins would disappear once the exercise began.

The Gurkhas were spread out in bunkers and other in-depth positions and they gave us the full volley when the attack was launched. Almost immediately, the runner arrived with fresh intelligence and orders. This time I paused, cleared my mind and thought hard before re-pointing my attack, diverting sections to where they were needed and, when the timing was right, call-ing up my reserves as the assault rolled forward. I gave very clear instructions; everyone knew their roles and played their part in a slickly exercised operation. By the time the sun had cleared the gorse-lined horizon, the attack was over, the Gurkha position taken. We'd done it. Leadership, teamwork and coolness under pressure had won the day.

There was no silent march back to the college on this occasion and I cut a much happier figure, standing tall, as we headed in for a clean-up and some hot food. Later, I went for my debrief with the OC – the major – and the hard-nosed training captain. In spite of the success, I was still expecting some sort of dressing down, or tepid compliment at best, but the officers were fulsome in their praise.

The training captain went out of his way to congratulate me, explaining he had treated me harder than the others on account of my greater experience. 'You arrived with a lot in your locker, so we were always going to have it in for you. But you did it. You rose to the challenge. You made massive progress over the four weeks.'

To my goggle-eyed surprise they told me I was very close to being awarded the prestigious Sword of Honour for that intake, but in the end they gave it to an outstanding young girl who had progressed the most. I said I had never been interested in accolades, which is true; for me it was about learning and developing, and that if they felt I had made good progress and was worthy of commission then that was honour enough for me. It was a good answer.

On the final day, the cadets formed up in brilliant sunshine outside the Old College for the famous Sovereign's Parade, the ceremonial flourish to celebrate our commission. Cadets are allowed to invite three guests and I chose my father and his parents. Standing to attention, eyes front, cupping the butt of my rifle, resplendent in my immaculate uniform with a single pip on the epaulette, I had never felt prouder. I had experienced that swelling of my heart several times in recent years, but this pride trumped all the others.

I was a 'one-pip wonder', a second lieutenant, the most junior officer. But I was an officer – a commissioned officer of the British Army. As I stood on the parade ground, face like granite in concentration, the Old College pillars gleaming in the bright sun, I needed discipline to suppress a smile. A thought had slipped into my head: *If only that copper who collared me outside WHSmith could be there to see me now.*

22

My mind had drifted towards suicidal thoughts from the moment I regained consciousness in hospital and I wasn't too worried about that. What's there to worry about if you are contemplating ending your life? You are seeing it as a release from an intolerable existence. If anything, knowing there's an opt-out clause, the fifth-floor option, keeps you going. I recognised that gloomy thoughts were going to be inevitable and, from time to time, my despair was going to slide towards the critical. I was always going to give my recovery every chance, but like all relationships, it's a two-way thing. It had to make an effort too. That's a fair deal.

What I didn't understand so well at first was the link between physical and mental health or, more accurately, the positive influence that good mental health can have on the physical. As a fitness freak, I had long understood the reverse – that regular, hard exercise induces a sense of well-being. But slowly, as my misery deepened and my wounds refused to heal, I made the connection. I realised it works the other way too. I am not qualified to explain how the happy chemicals like dopamine and serotonin influence cellular and vascular regeneration, so let's just call those chemical processes 'hope'. The bar of my hope levels didn't slide up and down the scale depending on the day and the mood. For months on end, it just sat at the bottom, occasionally twitching.

It was around the 15-month mark after my accident that the last residues of my hope began to drain away and I had my epiphany. It seems obvious now: my mood – the level of hope I felt

– had crashed and burned, and my wounds weren't healing. It was a vicious circle, or perhaps a catch-22 situation. To get better, I had to get happy, but to get happy, I had to be better. This sense of all hope slowly draining away continued to be dramatised in the vivid metaphor of my shower/torture sessions every other day. I was still being scrubbed, still howling with the pain, still watching my blood – the life blood – run out of my body, make a few turns around the plughole and disappear into the darkness underground. My imagination is not powerful enough to come up with a better representation of how perfectly that expressed how I was feeling in my soul. My painful life was literally and figuratively going down the drain. There it was for me every time I sat on that stool and the nurses/evil interrogators went to work on me with their soapy sponges and nail brushes/instruments of torture.

The infection was so persistent and aggressive that washing it off often failed to do the job and I had to be taken along to theatre to be debrided – scraped and grated clean. This happened about a dozen times and it was an horrendous experience every time. The surgeons had carried out the procedure many times in Orlando and thank God I had been in a coma. I lost so much blood on a few occasions that my life hung in the balance. When I came around in the recovery room, the all-over pain was so great I roared like a lion for hours, desperate for relief. I am not exaggerating whenever I say that this agony was every bit as intense as being on fire. It went on and on and on, for weeks and then months. If I was a boxer they would have stopped the fight in the twelfth but I was on round two hundred and something.

It was on a shower day that I had the lightbulb moment. Dignitas! Why the hell hadn't I thought of assisted suicide earlier? Get this whole nightmare over and done with, put me out of my misery and, in a separate way, put my family and friends out of theirs? As a parting charitable gift to society, by clearing off I'd also be saving the NHS and social security several million pounds. Doh! This was the best outcome for me, no question, and, once the initial grief had passed, probably for my family too. I was no longer going to be a burden and a worry to everyone for the rest of my days.

As for the wider world, well come on, was it really going to notice? Of course not. The world was going to get by just fine without me. I looked it up: over 150,000 people die every day. That's about 6,000 an hour, 100 a minute, drawing their last breath, felt their last heartbeat. We all croak, it's just a matter of when. My time had come. I'd had a cracking 33 years, a great last 15 or so at any rate. I had crammed more into those years than most would get into an active life of 250 years.

My existence had become intolerable, the future was an appalling prospect. I was worse than a waste of space, I was a mill-stone. My body and I had put up an epic fight but, well into the second year of it, I remained in agony and despair. So, I end my life. We're all winners. It's simple, it's lovely and neat, just as I like it. I hate mess, sloppy kit, and my life was one big crappy mess. When life's sergeant-major, making his inspection rounds, came to me, he wouldn't find a hole in my boots, some grit on my rifle and a loose strap on my Bergen. He'd find a man in utter disarray. His big moustache wouldn't be twitching, it would be bouncing up and done, his spittle drenching my face. 'Sort your shit out or fuck off out of here,' he'd be screaming. 'The world has no use for useless scumbag dossers like you, sonny boy!' I had no way of sorting out my shit, so the only option was to get the fuck out.

Many people, not least my loving, Christian mother, would argue with my decision, but frankly it's my life and I'll do with it as I please, thank you. Besides, a mother is not exactly going to say, *Phew, good plan, son. I've been waiting to hear those words for a while now. Glad you've finally seen sense. Bye, honey.* No, of course no one was going to encourage me along that route of thinking but that didn't mean people, deep down, weren't thinking my non-existence was not the worst idea. It was up to me to take responsibility for my own life. I had lived by that philosophy, now I was going to die by it.

Dignitas is a great institution in my book. If you have lost your life but not your mind, why shouldn't you have the option to end it all in a painless, thoughtful and caring manner with plenty of time to tidy up the loose ends and make those meaningful farewells? Most people just drop dead, or they die in a prolonged, tedious and sometimes agonising manner. The beauty of Dignitas, just as the name suggests, is that you can die with dignity. How many of us get to say goodbye to our loved ones in a controlled environment, maybe with a bit of ritual, a beautiful room, candles burning, some music playing in the background. You drink the cocktail of super-barbiturates and within ten minutes you're asleep, the heart slows steadily and then you slip away to the next world, or the darkness, whatever awaits. As far as deaths go, the assisted suicide arranged by Dignitas is top-of-the-range.

They handle the whole process very delicately and steadily. You don't just turn up in Switzerland, have a quick chat and get the injection, all sorted, one shot and you're in the ground. They are very thorough and they want to be absolutely certain that death is the right course of action. So, my correspondence with them, by email, went on for several months. It was so slow, in fact, that from time to time, my mind now set on it, I did consider the DIY version – a bottle of whisky in five minutes on top of a bunch of pills. But I couldn't bring myself to end it in such a messy fashion. It would have been too awful for my family, especially after all the care and love they had given me.

I spoke to the doctors about it and I spoke to Mum. She wasn't keen on the idea of driving me out to Switzerland so that I might die, then drive back with me on the passenger seat, a few handfuls of ashes in a nice urn. I needed someone to drive me out because I couldn't fly out and Dignitas insist on a bona fide friend or flesh-and-blood relative being present, at least to be in the building when it happens. But no one wanted to be an accessory to my death. That was deeply frustrating, but I got it. I could well imagine my own inner conflict if a mate asked me to do it for them. I'd try and talk them up about their recovery, about the life still to be led. I certainly wouldn't say, *Yeah, sure, no probs, mate. When do you want to go? I need to book off time from work.* It's a big call to assist someone in their death.

This was all going on in the winter months, me staring up at the dirty grey sky through the smeared condensation of my window. The news on the telly and the radio was nothing to cheer either. The world was in turmoil after the economic crash and the British Army was having a very hard time of it in Afghanistan, the casualty figures reported almost daily. I was becoming increasingly surly and aggressive to the people caring for me. I was an ugly person now, not the man I used to be, and I didn't blame the nurses for taking that much longer to answer my calls for attention. I wouldn't rush to help me either.

Some of the nurses had absolutely had enough of me and when they arrived to administer my meds, they handed them over in the paper cups and turned on their heel without a word. It was the same with the catering staff and my meals. They dumped the tray and fled. I was the monster in my lair and you got a snarl when you entered. I looked like a monster, I felt like a monster. It reached the point that Sister Adele came to tell me off, saying the staff would not tolerate my discourtesy any longer. I wasn't even very nice to my Mum, and if I thanked her at all for the lovely packed lunches she brought me in, I did so in the form of a bestial grunt. I lashed out at her sometimes too. I was told this was all part of the process for trauma victims, punishing those closest to you and caring for you – family and nurses – but it only made me hate myself more. I had become a perfect and revolting bastard.

I could never have foreseen how my outlook began to change. One day, Mum announced she had met someone through church who wanted to visit me. I shrugged and said, 'Whatever.' At this stage, strangers were preferable to friends and family. It didn't matter how aggressive and repulsive I was to them. I had just enough humanity left in me to recognise that my behaviour towards those who love and respect me – used to respect more like – was abhorrent and unacceptable. Strangers, fine. Bring them on. Good luck to them. (Besides, I had become so foul that most of my visitors had long since stopped coming. Mum was pretty well the only one left.)

The guy was an African pastor, she said, over here for a time, working in a parish in Oxford. He was called Billy. That's all she knew, but he was a good guy, not your regular preacher. For some reason, innate racism and ageism no doubt (more reason to hate myself), I was expecting an elderly white priest from South Africa. I was also expecting a dog collar and maybe a cross on a big chain. So, I was a little surprised when a middle-aged black guy in regular civvies walked into my room a few days later. I was even more surprised when he barely offered me a smile, more of a nod and a muttered hello. There was certainly no happy clapping. He parked himself in the armchair and our conversation, such as it was, proceeded in the form of staccato questions and grunts of affirmation or denial. (Him: 'So, your mum told me you're having a poor time of it.' Me: 'Yeah, that's about right.' ... Me: 'So, you're from Africa?' Him: 'Uh-huh.')

And so the conversation went on, barely a conversation at all, and with long periods of silence in between the grunts. I liked it. That was my kind of conversation for my mood: no pressure to be fucking chirpy. He was reserved, barely seemed interested. Maybe he'd seen a lot of suffering in his time and thought little of it these days. *Suffering? What's the big deal? It's everywhere, my friend.* That was the vibe he gave off. He didn't tell me to stop feeling sorry for myself or anything like it. He had an aura of kindness about him, the undemonstrative version that you sense and doesn't need to be spelt out in words or actions. He must have been a man of great kindness because why else would he go to the big effort of coming to sit in the company of an angry, messed up stranger?

After an hour or so, he got up, looking as bored as he had when he arrived, and said: 'Okay, I better go and get my train. I've enjoyed meeting you.'

I said: 'Yeah, I enjoyed it too. It was good of you to come.' That was just about the nicest thing I had said to anyone in months, *Go fuck yourself* being about the second nicest.

He said: 'You want me to come back?'

I could hardly say *no* and, actually, I wanted him to come back, so I said, 'Yeah, that would be great. What's your name by the way?'

'Billy. Pastor Billy, that'll do. Just call me that.'

'Okay, Pastor Billy, thanks. See you whenever. I'll be here. I won't be going anywhere.'

He gave me his first smile and walked out.

So, Pastor Billy came back the following week and the week following and the one after that. He came five times in all, and I was pleased to see him every time. We talked a little more each time, about nothing in particular. He never asked me about my accident and I never offered to tell him. At first, I had been keen to share the experience with my visitors but I soon tired of trotting it out over and over. Pastor Billy may have been interested in the details, I don't know. All he needed to know was that I was in a bad place in my head and in my soul. He didn't have to tell me that's why he was at my bedside. Why else would he bother coming?

The kindness of strangers is a wonderful thing. We've probably all had that thrill of gratitude and connection when someone runs after us in the street handing back the wallet or keys we've dropped. We go on our way, feeling a little better about the day, our faith in humanity restored or enhanced. I had that feeling in a major way with Pastor Billy, this stranger from Africa who owed me nothing, just coming to sit with me in my suffering, not say too much, just connect, just be there for me. I well up a little when I think of Pastor Billy now and I wonder what on earth he is up to, what other stricken soul he is ministering to in his calm and humble fashion. Some religious people really like to show you they are good, caring people. It's a form of grandstanding, power games almost. *Hey, look how good I am!* Not Pastor Billy. He was just a regular good guy who gave a fig for other people.

On the third or fourth visit, I felt so comfortable with him – I actually looked forward to his visits – I told him my plans to end my life and that I was some way down the line of the process with Dignitas. I explained that none of my friends or family were prepared to drive me out and assist my suicide. I was nervous about telling him, a devout Christian, and he sat listening to me, hands in prayer position under his chin, his brow furrowed. When I was done, still deep in thought, he got up to leave and said he'd give it some thought. He said it neutrally, just like he said everything, like he was weighing up whether to have tea or coffee.

He hadn't ruled it out on the spot but I was anxious on the morning of his next visit. He came in, eased himself into the armchair and said, 'Yeah, no problem, I'll drive you to Switzerland and see you through it.'

'Really?' I hadn't felt so thrilled – well, since the wheels left the runway and I rose into the clear blue sky that fateful morning. 'You're serious? You'll do it?'

'Yes, I will, Jamie. I understand. I want to help people in their suffering. But I'll do it on one condition.'

'Fine, anything. Tell me.'

'That you wait a month.'

'Why? Why a month? Let's just get on with it. I've made my decision. Why hang about?'

My anger was never far from the surface at this time, and I felt it about to burst like one of my pustulant boils.

'That's my condition, Jamie. Take it or leave it.'

It was the best offer I was going to get, probably the only one. I offered him my hand – the one on the end of the Hitler salute, and we shook.

'A month it is.'

'A month it is.'

* * *

It's amazing how the prospect of imminent death can raise the spirits. Immediately following the pact with Pastor Billy, my mood brightened and the heaviness that had enveloped my soul like a heavy toxic fog began to clear. I had forgotten what happiness felt like and I guess that's the deal with happiness, it felt good. I wasn't cracking jokes and playing air drums to the radio, but I was smiling a little and I had that constant, physical sensation of excitement that I used to get ahead of an adventure to an exotic location. The following morning nurses who had grown so wary of me were visibly surprised to be greeted with courtesy and gratitude. That made me feel even better about myself, about the world, treating these hard-working poorly paid carers with the respect they so richly deserved. Christ, I was almost human. Thanks to death, it was great to be alive. I even started enjoying Steve Wright on the radio. You're all right, Steve!

A few days after Billy had left for his parish, the surgeon, Mr Ghosh, came to visit me. He too was in buoyant mood, thrilled to inform me that rolls of fresh cadaver skin were on their way to Stoke Mandeville, enough to carry out a huge grafting operation to my back, upper right flank and scalp. The miraculous antidepressant effects of death! Everyone was on a high. It's a peculiar world you have entered when the despair of one man's death becomes another man's joy. It's strange too to discover and live in this world where skin is a commodity, a product, harvested and transported up and down the country like fruit and veg, sold by surgeons, and paid for in gratitude. Even stranger that wearing a dead man's skin, the skin of a pig even, no longer excited feelings of revulsion but of happiness.

I had come to dread these grafts and the unbearable pain they brought, and I can't say I punched the air when Ghosh scheduled the procedure. But I felt indifferent about it. I wasn't bothered. What did it matter? I was going to be shaking around in a little ceramic urn soon, so what's another few days of agony? Besides, it may make the long road journey to Switzerland that little less uncomfortable. It was a long operation and, as usual, I screamed like a baby when I awoke in the recovery room. Somehow the pain wasn't quite as intense as after previous grafts and, back in my room, I didn't freefall back into the darkness. Was this my body's chemical response to optimism, the dopamine and serotonin streaming out of my glands?

About five days later, when the pain began to settle, I noticed a distinct difference in my body. It's difficult to describe, but I knew before they removed the dressings to clean the donor sites that some sort of change had occurred. When the nurses peeled off the bandages and the gauze, I didn't yelp, sob and protest quite as volubly as normal (this regular procedure was no pain picnic either). As the nurses carefully removed the layers of pussy and bloody dressing, dropping them into the big pedal bin, they became increasingly chipper and chatty, amazed by what they were seeing.

'These have taken beautifully, Jamie,' one of them gushed. 'He's done a fine job on you, that Mr Ghosh.'

I am sure he had done a fine job because he is a fine plastic surgeon, but I knew the greater truth. The skin had taken and was healing fast because my mind was flooding my body with happy chemicals and hormones. I was getting better – and it was all because I knew I was going to die and the misery and pain were going to be over.

I am not a religious man but I have tried to see the light over the years, just never quite managed the leap of faith required. Is that not the meaning of faith? To believe in something of which there is no hard proof. To believe in something that exists before your very eyes is just to know a fact. It's right there, plain as a pikestaff, easy to believe in. But to believe in something that you cannot see or know, that's faith – and, ever the pragmatist, I had always struggled to engage with an unknowable quantity.

But, in these days and weeks after the pact, seeing my skin healing before my very eyes, I was experiencing some sort of low-grade religious experience. At the very least, it was a sense of tremendous wonder. If that wonder was stirred only by observing the power of nature, watching the active connection between mind, body and soul, then it was still wonder. The word 'miracle' was working its way around my mind and when the nurses and doctors and visitors came to see me, the word was even being uttered in one form or another. 'Why, it's miraculous, Jamie!'

As I lay there, still in great pain but not as much, still in a gloom but grey not pitch black, Pastor Billy hovered in the atmosphere, a black angel above my head. He had triggered the reversal, this quiet, kind man from Africa whose country of origin I didn't know, whose surname I didn't know! This stranger turns up at my side, at the lowest point in my life when, night and day, I had begun to dream of death, the only release from the torment. This man of God who never spoke to me of God, was he my guardian angel come to save me? He was most certainly an intervention, but could he really be divine, or at least sent by the divine? He said he prayed for me all the time and on each visit, asking my permission first, he said one short prayer over me, but that was it. Otherwise, he never raised the matter of faith, his or mine. Perhaps he was just very astute and suspected, rightly, that I would have barked him into the nurses' station if he came over all pious and righteous on me, telling me to repent my sins or feel the flames of hell on my skin. But why did he come? Why me?

He wasn't my first angel. The two guys who kept shouting at me, for fully 20 minutes, to stay alive before the casevac chopper arrived – what about them? Were they angels? They succeeded in keeping me from sliding into an unconsciousness from which I would never emerge. They probably saved my life (for better or for worse). Yes, they were angels of a sort. And then there was Renee, the lovely Renee with her honeyed voice. She was an angel, no question, but I slightly fancied her and that didn't feel quite right. You're not meant to get passionate and tender about angels, but it was hard not to dream about her and she continued to be a big presence in my life back in England, a vivid imaginative presence. Now, Pastor Billy! I was beginning to wonder if perhaps someone *was* watching over me after all.

Three weeks after our pact, Pastor Billy made another appearance. He had never said when he was coming back. He came in, barely even saying hello, just muttering his greetings as always, and dropped into the armchair, hands in prayer under his chin. As before, we spoke in bursts, skirting around the state of my health and the state of mind and soul, not mentioning God or Jesus Christ or faith. We were like two guys on a train occasionally looking up from our papers to pass the time of day. As before, I found his presence deeply calming. It's fair to say that since regaining consciousness he had been the only person with whom I made a true connection, and I had missed him since his last visit.

When the time came, he levered himself to his feet and asked my permission to say his prayer over me. He closed his eyes, clasped his hands together, bowed his head and, barely audible, muttered his devotions.

'I guess we should fix that date for our trip to Switzerland,' he said, and made his way towards the door. 'It'll be a month next week.'

When he turned around, I said, 'Actually, Pastor Billy, I've been thinking. I don't want to die any longer. I want to live.'

A huge toothy smile spread from one ear to the other. I had seen him smile a couple of times in the past, but not like this.

He slapped the frame of the door and said, 'Okay, well, I'll be seeing you then, Jamie.' That's what he always said when he left.

But I never saw him again.

23

Once a year, the Cambridge OTC rolled out the red carpet for its cadets and honourable guests, a bit of swank between the sweat, the combat jackets swapped for dinner jackets. In the spring of 2003, the grand evening took place in the august surroundings of King's College, founded in 1441 by Henry VI. High-profile brass, including the Chief of the General Staff, attended the event, and each cadet was assigned a dignitary to chaperone. I was placed next to a very interesting character who, it soon became clear, was the training major of 21 SAS, the reservist battalion of Britain's elite Special Forces regiment. From the way the conversation unrolled, I was aware that the seating plan that evening was no accident.

For some time now, both my commanding officer and the Regimental Sergeant Major at the Cambridge OTC had been pressing me to go for Special Forces Selection – the long, gruelling process, the only one – by which a promising young soldier, officer or other ranks, can get to pull on the famous sandy beret of the Special Air Service. I had developed huge respect for both men. When they talked, I listened. I was, they told me, exhausting every challenge the OTC could throw at me. Assuming I completed 'P' Company, there was only one major trial left to be conquered. Flattered, I had given the prospect some thought, but parked it at the back of my mind. The first phase of Selection was a year-long commitment, and I had the Para course to focus on – and maybe Sandhurst too – and then my university finals at the end of the academic year. That was enough even for my greedy appetite for life.

I listened attentively to my guest for the evening and, as the courses came and went, the major quietly went about weaving his magic. His inspirational tales of the achievement to be cherished, pushing oneself further than ever before, worked their way into my highly motivated and competitive nature. The major's blandishments had a similar effect on me as the flutter of a red rag and a spear in the side of an already furious bull. By the time the port was making its circuit of the linen table, I had resolved to go for it.

I had read all the great books about the SAS from the regiment's foundation in the Second World War; I had heard all the anecdotes passed down the military grapevine. Making my way back to Norwich that evening, my mind swarmed. Could I really see myself as a member of that mythical institution, the spearhead tip of the British Army? Was I getting above myself? What if I failed – how would that affect my confidence? What about my studies?

The doubts re-formed and massed but the tenacious, bloody-minded element of my nature mounted a concerted counterattack. Could I ever have imagined completing a Cambrian? Could I ever have foreseen myself signing up for 'P' Company, one of the hardest training courses in world military? No, but I did. Could I ever have imagined getting a place at a good university? No, but I did. Could I ever have imagined mastering four difficult languages? No, but I did. Could I ever have pictured myself arriving at Sandhurst to become a commissioned officer? No, but I was about to give that a crack too. So, I asked myself, what am I frightened of? If I failed, I failed – and if I did, it wasn't going to be for lack of character. The next morning, I rang the RSM and asked for my name to be put forward.

The first phase began in the autumn term, not long after my return from Sandhurst. One evening every week, I took a train to London and walked up to the barracks for my instruction. It was not what I had imagined. The basic fitness tests were no great challenge for a man who had passed 'P' Company and the rest of the time was spent in a classroom studying maps and taking notes. Map reading, I was told, was a black art, probably the most important skill I would learn to carry out my role effectively. The aim was for a candidate to be able to look at a map and instantly compute the terrain and topography so clearly that the mind's eye was effectively seeing the land in 3D and aerial all at once.

That mastered, the course got serious. Basic fitness turned into beasting. You don't need a large space to run a man into the ground and the empty car park of the barracks was all the senior 'badge' of our intake needed to leave his men gasping and sodden by the time he was done with them. By Christmas, a handful decided that the effort was not for them and dropped out.

There was nothing mysterious, nothing magical, nothing superhuman about what we were doing. It was just maps and fitness. It was even a bit boring. All they wanted to know is whether the candidate was going to be an asset. Could the guy cut it? Part of proving that worthiness was just turning up week in, week out, sitting in a classroom poring over maps, learning arcane terms of topography like 'azimuth' and 're-entrant', and then heading outside and letting an aggressive man shout them up and down tarmac to the point of collapse. Then come back for more of the same the following week.

It is no secret that the hardest training in the British Army takes place in the Brecon Beacons of Wales, just over the Herefordshire border. That's where I soon started spending alternate weekends as the graded course moved up a level of difficulty. The

Cambridge contingent of the 138-strong intake met at the OTC HQ on Friday afternoon and, at the start, it took two minibuses to transport all the hopefuls to their remote and spartan camp in the wilds of Wales.

The first weekend, we just walked for two days, getting familiar with the terrain, the landmarks and the rapidly changeable, often severe weather. I remembered the difficulty of it only too well from the Cambrians. We were escorted in smaller groups by a senior badge alerting us to the topographical features we had studied in the classroom, a spur here, a saddle there, up a convex slope, down a concave one. So far, so easy, pleasant almost.

The selection process is step-by-step, steady and meticulous, slowly scaling the contours of the challenge. It's not crazy-intense like 'P' Company, flat out for three weeks. At least not in the early stages. The marches became harder as the fortnights went by. I was enjoying the range of characters I met: surgeons, bricklayers, teachers, financial analysts, lawyers, serving officers, NCOs and privates. It was the ultimate leveller, no privileges, no special treatment, no favouritism. The course leaders didn't give a shit who we were. They were interested only in whether a candidate had the fitness, the resilience and the personality to perform at the highest level of military operations.

Every fortnight, the group shed a cluster of candidates, leaving an ever-shrinking hardcore to push on. There was no way I was going to 'VW' – the slang they used for voluntary withdrawal. If I collapsed, fine, but I wasn't going to slink away because it was too hard. The decreasing size of the group on the forced marches reflected the progress being made. The smaller the unit became, the harder the challenges that lay ahead, until finally the candidates were ready to head out on their own. About a third of the contenders were left at this point, when the challenge moved beyond a test of mere fitness and endurance. Navigating the route alone, no one to offer help or encouragement, it would become a test of character, clear thinking and composure under pressure.

The Endurance or 'Hills phase' of Selection culminates in Test Week. To qualify, candidates must first complete a 16-mile march over Pen-y-fan – the highest mountain in the Brecons. They carry full kit and they must complete the task in under four hours, whatever the weather. After that, they are subjected to the most rigorous medical examination in the Armed Forces. Only Special Forces and fighter pilots are obliged to meet the standards.

It was high summer of 2004 and I had graduated from university when I turned up at the OTC depot for the final trip to the Welsh mountains. Where once there had been two full minibuses from Cambridge, there was now only one and it was less than half full. We could have squeezed into a car.

Test Week is a compressed and intensified version of the marches they had conducted over the previous six months. Every march of Test Week gets harder and harder, each one double the length of the standard tests completed by regular units. The distance covered increases every day, the weight carried every two. All marches are solitary exercises, all having to be completed within stringent time limits.

What remained of the original intake contracted gradually over the week. By the final day, only about two dozen were still in the running. I was doing okay. I was strong on 'nav' so I never got lost, I was naturally fit and I was stronger than my slight build suggested. (If I was next to you in a supermarket queue, you'd never guess I was an elite soldier.)

'P' Company, I found, had been harder physically, but Selection was much tougher in other ways. I was learning to be a thinking soldier. I was on my own, no moral or physical support, on the move constantly and at pace, mostly in the dark, against the clock. The mental pressure was huge, thinking on my feet, lungs heaving, sweat pouring, map shaking in my hand under the light of my wobbling head torch. Just one miscalculation would send me the wrong route and I'd have blown my chances. By the time I corrected myself, too much time would have passed, too much precious energy expended. All that effort over the year would have been for nothing. One strike and I was out.

The week ends with a 40-miler known as 'The Long Drag'. It was midnight and I had had four hours sleep when the lights of my barracks block flashed on. After a week of marches, every muscle in my body ached, especially in the legs. Immediately, we all set about our daily remedial tasks, using rolls of medical tape to seal up the welts on each other's backs and shoulders, shredded raw by the weight of our bouncing Bergens. For the blisters on my feet and ankles, I applied gel plasters and wrapped them in zinc oxide tape.

It was pitch dark and there was a heavy mist when we assembled on the parade square for roll call and then climbed into the back of the four-tonne canvas-topped Bedfords for the drive back out. My dry pack weight had been increased to 55 pounds, plus food (lots), water (lots), webbing and weapon, for a total of 80 pounds. To pass, I was going to have to carry that for 40 miles over the hills and across the bogland in under 20 hours.

It was cold and damp when I was dropped on the western side of the Brecons and disappeared into the darkness. The mist cleared, burned off by the sun, and the greater visibility came as a huge relief. Being unable to see the end of your nose is no aid to navigation. But the climbing sun brought different problems and by noon, about seven hours in, it was blistering hot, adding to the agonising pain I was in. My feet had burst open in several places, the dressings had slid off under the remorseless tread of my boots.

The pain of my raw skin, rubbing with every step, became so great that it was almost impossible to move and, limping into the halfway stage I was only too happy to accept the medic's offer of Tylex painkillers. There were still 20 miles to go in the intense afternoon heat but the 'smarties' – a mixture of codeine and paracetamol – kicked in quickly and soon I was eating up the terrain as fast as my body was eating up the calories. Over the course of the run, I wolfed 12 Ginsters pasties, 16 Snickers bars, 8 rolls rammed with meat and cheese, and drank 2 litres of water every hour. My accelerated metabolism obliged to me to pull over three times to take an 'elephant dump' in the bushes. Ten miles from the finish I took a second dose of painkillers and powered on, knowing I was going to make it with time to spare. In the event, as the last of the sun sunk over the Cray Reservoir, I crossed the line 2 hours inside the cut-off in an impressive 18 hours flat.

I was elated and then, almost immediately, delirious. I remember being directed to a stores truck and filling my face with snacks and gulping energy drinks. After that, it became something of a blur. Two medics carried me to the back of a soft-top Land Rover, laid me down, slapping my face to keep me conscious. By the time we reached the medical centre back at the camp, heat stress, or hyperthermia, had set in and I was shaking uncontrollably.

My knees giving out, I was laid on the floor and the medics wriggled me into an emergency bivvy bag and sunk a fluid drip into each arm. The fluid bags were replaced regularly, and at four in the morning I was woken from a profound sleep, my bladder at bursting point. I called out and two medics helped me up, my feet so swollen that every step was excruciating, and I almost gave up and pissed on the floor.

Over the 18 hours of the march, I had eaten the equivalent of three days of meals, but my body was still ravenous for energy and replenishment. The best the medic could muster was a box of cold fish and chips. Nothing had ever tasted so delicious and, when I was done, I finished a second straight off and washed it down with a litre bottle of Gatorade, the fluid and saline drips still hanging out of my arms. No sooner had I swallowed the last mouthful then I was out for the count again and stayed that way for six hours until I was shaken awake and told it was breakfast. I made my way over to the cookhouse, hobbling and grabbing any support to hand, and I sat down to the largest cooked breakfast I had ever seen, let alone eaten.

A coach took us to a service station on the M4 where the RSM from Cambridge was waiting with the minibus. Of the five of us from the OTC who had made it to Test Week, I was the only one to pass. I was one of only a fraction of the original intake still standing – and only just. It would be over a week before I walked normally again and a fortnight before I attempted any form of exercise.

Of all the contenders, I was neither the fastest, the strongest or the sharpest, but I was one of the gutsiest, I reckon. I was a solid all-rounder who never gave up. I had proved my resilience and character and shown I had the 'animal cunning' to survive extreme conditions in the wild. All successful candidates probably had a bit of that cunning and when I thought about it after the event, I came to understand that my tough teenage years were not the great catastrophe I had come to regard them. Yes, they were tough years, but they had at least made me resourceful and streetwise. From the age of 12, I was forced to cope by myself, to be savvy, to get by without the assistance of others. And that's exactly what the UK's elite regiment was looking for.

Over the year that followed, based back at home with my mother in Leighton Buzzard, I went off to complete the subsequent phases of Special Forces training. It wasn't easy and there was a great deal of technical detail to master, but very few who have passed the Hills phase stumble and fail. When the final exercise was over, we were bussed to a camp in the Midlands. There was an at-ease parade, but absolutely no ceremony. The commanding officer made a short no-frills speech, congratulating us on our achievement and welcoming us to the SAS. 'Well done, you're all badged' was about the long and short of it. All the seniors from the course were present and I was touched to see the proud face of my Directing Staff (DS) from Cambridge in the gathering. He'd been a great source of encouragement and support throughout. A sergeant handed me the famous sandy beret with the winged dagger badge and I worked it over my scalp.

Collecting my kit, I paused to look at myself in the mirror. Finally, I allowed the pride to balloon inside my chest. My education as a man was over. My life could now begin.

24

I was discharged from Stoke Mandeville in August 2009, almost exactly two years from the day my aircraft caught fire, eighteen months after my 'discharge' from Chelmsford and about nine months after Pastor Billy's intervention – or visitation, transformative kindness, call it what you like. Perhaps it was the meds, perhaps it was because he didn't speak that much that I can remember so little about this strange man who came to visit me on half-a-dozen occasions. I didn't get to know *him* at all. His character was elusive, insubstantial, ethereal. He passed through my life like a good ghost, a holy spirit, rescued me from hell and vanished. It wasn't the case that the day after he left I woke up and discovered I had turned into a stand-up comedian and a saint. I was still depressed, fearful, frustrated and grouchy. But I had changed, no question, and all I know now is that there has not been a moment since my last encounter with Pastor Billy when I have contemplated again the idea of taking my own life. Yes, I have had many dark days and felt utterly miserable, but from the day he wafted out of my life I have been determined to give life a go, to make the most of what I had been left with.

Prior to being discharged, the tedious routine of daily life continued, every day virtually the same as the one that preceded it and the one I saw coming. Only a change in the sky through the square of window to my right gave any sense of a changing world. The nurse came in about seven, slapped on the blood pressure cuff, gave me some painkillers in a paper cup and yanked back the curtains. I pressed the button on the handheld control, raising the top half of my bed so that I was sitting upright. That always gave me a childish thrill. The second excitement of the day was breakfast. I always had Marmite on toast with extra butter because I understood enough about nutrition to know that my depleted body would welcome a surfeit of healthy fats. In the army, I had learned to listen to my body, to work out what it wanted for the task in hand.

I grew tired of watching the news. Current affairs tended to drag down my mood, and the breakfast presenters had a little too much chirp for my liking. They seemed almost delighted to inform viewers that the world had gone into economic melt-down and that two more soldiers had been killed by a roadside bomb. So, most days, I just stared at the ceiling for an hour or so, daydreamed and made plans about how to adapt to the new life awaiting me on the outside. Otherwise, I'd sleep, listen to some music from my iPod in its docking station, trawl the internet and, if my brain was feeling lively enough, read a book. It was often a Terry Pratchett because I liked being transported into a fantasy world far removed from my grey reality. Reading was hard, though, because I only had one working arm, the other still paying its respects to Hitler and the Nazis. I was drowsy most of the time, too, from the meds and the lack of physical and mental stimulation.

My wound dressings were changed every other day and I always dreaded the moment. Even though the nurses were work-ing on ever-decreasing areas of unhealed skin, the pain remained constant. (There is no difference in pain levels between a small and big cut on your fingertip.) The arrival of the physios every day was an event, I suppose. It was action of sorts, and it gave me a small sense of progress to squeeze the rubber balls and play with the other toys. My condition was improving by barely noticeable degrees but after a time I was strong enough to be wheeled once in a while to the physio centre at the far end of the hospital, where I did a little bit of cardio, mostly on a bike as the physios were trying to strengthen my legs.

On other days, I'd practise my walking, shuffling up and down draughty corridors in my open-backed gown. Any form of exercise, no matter how insignificant, was shattering and after lunch I always fell into a heavy sleep and often didn't wake up till Mum came to visit around teatime. When the effort of going to the toilet five yards away was too much, I used to manoeuvre my legs out and lean against the bed. My kidneys were working well again and, eager to stay hydrated and flush out all the toxins from my meds, I was drinking water by the litre and pissing so copiously that the bottle often overflowed and the nurses would have to come and mop the floor. I wasn't giving them many opportunities to fall in love with me.

I desperately wanted to get on with rebuilding my life but when I was finally discharged, it was not the joyful occasion I had imagined. Institutionalised and bedbound for so long – two years of my life in a bed! – the day loomed darkly on the horizon. This was partly because I was a long way from being fit and well. My wounds had still not healed, I was still going to be rooted to a mattress, it was going to be months before I could negotiate the stairs, and Mum and I were going to be living cheek-by-jowl in the only downstairs room apart from the galley kitchen.

It may well have been the sheer boredom of my existence, coupled with the growing urgency to give Mum a break and some time to herself, but I began to force myself outside. At first, I would just stand in the postage-stamp garden, breathing the fresh air and, if I was lucky, watch a blackbird pluck a worm from the small square of grass. For a change of scene, I went out the front door and stood on the drive. After a time, I began walking the ten metres to the end and back. We lived in a small cul-de-sac made up of ten semi-detached homes, but the prospect of walking the length of it felt filled me with the same awe and trepidation as an expedition through the Hindu Kush. To complete a lap of it became my next goal and I was determined to do the 150 yards, unaided. I was forced to abandon the first few attempts, turning back halfway, dizzy and short of breath and convinced I was going to going to crash to the asphalt. There was also an element of stage fright because the curtains were twitching with curious neighbours eager for a glimpse of the Frankenstein's monster living in their midst.

It was a couple of weeks before I nailed the achievement and I celebrated with a three-hour sleep. I woke with aching limbs, like I had completed Special Forces Selection all over again. Slowly, I built up my strength and confidence and an indifference to my audience. Still walking and shuffling with baby steps, I started to up the number of laps, pushing to complete one more every other day or so. Round and round I went, day after day, week after week, no faster than a man in his nineties.

By winter, I was ready to venture out of the cul-de-sac. Again, it was boredom, the lust for adventure, that drove me on. My limited strength and walking ability had determined the boundaries of my confinement, but I was also scared to show my face. It was very swollen, very red and very scarred, my scalp likewise. I had only a few tufts of hair and my ears were mangled stubs. I felt profoundly self-conscious and, inevitably, people gawped at me. A passer-by would startle on catching a glimpse of me and look away like they'd been slapped. I was safe from this in the cul-de-sac by and large but the next road, a short stone's throw away, was another world altogether. It was a very quiet residential street, but it had moving cars and moving people on it, and that terrified me.

The day I made it all the way to the newsagent I still look upon as one of the great achievements of my life. It wasn't so much the distance I covered – about 600 yards in all – it was buying the paper. I stood outside composing myself with deep breaths, hobbled in, picked out my newspaper and looked the shop owner in the eye – like I was no different to any other customer. He gave me a big smile and dropped the change in my hand – like I was no different to any other customer. It was a curiously emotional experience but the tears I felt welling on my shuffle home were tears of happiness and relief. I was half-expecting him to screw up his face and say, 'Ugh!'

Building some resilience to this pathetic, debilitating self-consciousness, I had a wonderful breakthrough moment sitting in the doctor's surgery one morning. The waiting room was deathly silent, as they always are, pregnant with that strange tension, no one quite sure of the gravity of the others' condition. A very young girl was staring at me, inquisitive not horrified. She was standing between her mother's legs there twisting on the spot with a finger to her lips, her eyes locked on me, her brow furrowed. After a time, she turned to her Mum and, very loudly, asked, 'Mummy, what's wrong with that man's face?' Her mother went puce and whispered in her ear, but I leaned forward and said, 'It's okay. Shall I tell you what happened?' And, sparing her the gory details, I did. The girl was very sweet and asked me a few questions and told me it must have been very sore and that I must have been super brave.

Kids are bloody great. I learned that during those early days of my recovery. They never looked away in embarrassment. Often, they would stare and stare but without prejudice, just pure fasci-nation, their little minds trying to model the story that may have led to me looking as I did. Children in the age group from about eight years old to mid-teens were the least likely to look away and it was from them I was most likely to receive a genuinely lovely, unembarrassed smile. No grown-up ever stared – nor would I – but reactions differed and soon I reckoned I could tell someone's character in the flash of their glance at me. Some instantly flashed a smile, a few screwed up their face in disgust, but most were horrified and upset, unable to form a coherent response in their facial expressions and I knew they would be at a loss for words if we stopped to talk. That inability to discuss the Elephant Man in the room was something I'd get used to.

My appearance wasn't helped by my shambolic baggy clothing. I looked as though I had emerged from beneath a railway arch after a meths bender, and my walk and posture would have scored pretty low on *Strictly Coming Dancing*. I'd had to develop a high knee lift, utilising the thigh muscles, to compensate for what they call the 'bilateral foot drop' caused by the removal of my shin muscles. I walked a little like a show pony with shin splints. I was also hunched forward Quasimodo-style, owing to the contracture of my skin, the absence of abdominal muscles and, unknown to me at the time, the growth of a massive hernia.

With a walking stick in my left hand and my right arm stuck halfway in the Nazi salute, it was no wonder I drew attention to myself. Certainly, no one would have thrown me a look, and thought, *Hey, look there goes another fully badged trooper with 21 SAS!* That said, some good people used to stop me and ask if I was in the Armed Forces. The heavy sacrifice of our troops in Afghanistan was major news at the time and there was a good deal of public awareness and sympathy for the wounded. Some, I figured, probably thought I was a veteran suffering from PTSD and might bite their heads off, and that was the reason why they looked away and hurried along.

For almost a year, I left Leighton Buzzard only to go to hospital for a procedure or a check-up with the plastic surgeons.

I treated myself as a case study in a long-term project, chalking up my progress in tiny incremental grades. I upped the distances I walked, and I set myself small tasks each day. I could never have imagined the day that making a cup of tea would bring such a sense of achievement. Getting up to find the remote control rather than shouting for Mum, reading for an hour without falling asleep, going out to fetch a pint of milk – these were the milestones by which I was able to see that my life was improving.

In a way, my life was a Lilliputian version of my life in the Armed Forces. Once I had come to see my achievements in a context, I was able to congratulate myself and even feel a little pride in the execution of tasks or tests of endurance. In this peculiar world, going to Tesco and coming back with a bag of groceries left me as exhausted as a Cambrian Patrol and, coming through it, not giving up, gave me every bit as much satisfaction. I was healing mentally – or spiritually – as much as physically. I was learning to cope. I wasn't happy but my resilience and my morale were growing. I had a very long way to go and some tough operations awaiting me, but I was not going to be defeated. I am not a patient man, but I am always happy to learn new skills. Over that year, I took the first steps in learning the virtue of patience.

The vicious vortex that had swept me down and down to the darkest depths was switching direction. The condition of my skin was a good metaphor, an outward representation, of how I was feeling inside. Those states of being, the physical and the mental, were very closely bound and they were healing at roughly the same rate. That may have been a coincidence, but I doubt it. You could make a fairly accurate estimate of my happiness levels by the state of my very slowly healing skin. With every inch that sealed over, there was a barely perceptible but commensurate inflation of my buoyancy.

The growth of hope was not vigorous; it didn't shoot skywards, it grew with the stately leisure of an oak tree, taking its time, growing strong roots. The great thing about hope is that it's self-feeding. The more hope I felt, the less I had to look to others or to external sources of stimulation for the nourishment and support needed to sustain my evolution as a new being. Gradually, this gave Mum the greater freedom and the greater peace of mind she so desperately needed and deserved. My accident had been as much a life-changing experience for her as me and she was having to dig very deep every day to cope with the hideous challenge that life had thrown at her.

Having a tidy mind, a love of order, helped too. I began laying out plans and goals and charting my progress with a daily schedule, like I was a master builder overseeing the construction of a dwelling from the ground up. When I placed a tick next to 'Make cup of tea' or 'buy Mum chocolates' I was able to see the physical evidence of my efforts – a fresh brew or Mum's smile – and move on to the next satisfying task. My rise from the dust of my shattered life was slow and you'd only notice the difference if you came to see me every few weeks. It was a few bricks at a time, the fixtures and fittings still a long way down the schedule of works.

I began to accept that I was never going to be the guy I once was, and the more I let go, the easier it became to imagine a different future. I committed to developing another version of myself, like a new generation of software – Jamie Hull 3.0 in my case – and I tried to persuade myself that, once I got used to the updates, I could grow to like and perhaps even admire myself for a different set of features and tricks. Quite what that version was going to look like I couldn't yet say, but part of the adventure – there was always adventure! – was going to be in the discovery of it.

An example of this came from the daily exercise I was taking. My walks became ever-increasing circles, fanning out from surrounding streets into the town centre and when spring came, up into the beautiful hills around Leighton Buzzard. By the start of summer, I was completing circuits on the wooded paths of the Dunstable Downs, coming back exhausted and ravenous, but with a powerful sense of achievement and something that was starting to resemble the outline of happiness. The more I walked, the more I ate and the more fuel I put in my body, and the stronger my heart and muscles became, the closer I edged towards restoration.

Almost three years on from the flames, some areas of my skin remained unhealed – mainly my uppermost body and scalp – but the agony had been downgraded to acute pain, my mobility had increased markedly and I was able to see into the future with a little more clarity and confidence. Once I had been a good middle- and long-distance runner. Those days were now over, but as I bounced along the country lanes in my new funny way of walking, I dreamed of becoming a hiker and started planning trips to the Yorkshire Dales, the Lake District and the Alps. The drive was still there, it was coming back, but the goals had changed.

Reflecting on these early days of recovery, I should stress that I was no Zebedee, bouncing with glee from one task to the next. I was still very much down in the dumps, still more of an Eeyore character, gloomy and pessimistic and highly unlikely to beam sunshine into your day. If you were unlucky enough to find yourself in my presence, sure, you will have felt a mixture of sympathy and horror, you may have been impressed by my fortitude and resilience, and you may even have chuckled at some dark humour, but you certainly wouldn't have left my company with a frisky shake of the tail and a spring in your step.

I had made little to no effort to see or even contact my friends since my discharge. I didn't want a social life. I was in a survivalist state-of-mind and there was no room in my bunker for others. I was angry, quick-tempered and bloody-minded, resentful of other people's happiness and capabilities. I may not have hated the sight of you, and I may even have greeted you with a corner-of-the-mouth smile, but I'd be growling and griping at you soon enough.

I was furious with Fate. I had done so much to turn my life around. Since my errant teenage years, I don't believe I could have done any more to transform myself into a figure worthy of respect and perhaps, from time to time, admiration. I was seething that all my efforts had been hurled down in flames.

Then, the phone rang. It was my old mate Pete Mash from Colorado.

25

... Or Dr Peter Mash to give him his full title. Pete was a senior with the Cambridge University OTC when I joined the corps. By day, he was studying Engineering at Emmanuel College. By evening and weekends, he was an OTC devotee, barmy about the army and mulling a career as a regular. In one of my first outings, he was the instructor on the map-reading course and instantly I fell under the spell of his cheerful enthusiasm. He has brains coming out of his ears and, if you could bottle his energy, he would put Red Bull out of business overnight. He went for Selection, only failing in the last stages, just before Test Week, owing to a medical problem. That was a shame because he is a highly capable, ballsy character and his zest for life is infectious, his appetite for challenges insatiable. He is also highly practical and will not be beaten by a technical challenge. (The SAS instructors called him 'The Professor'.) We quickly became good mates and, although I went my way and he went to the States soon after Cambridge, our friendship endured.

Pete was working in Colorado Springs when he called, running his own company, Light Blue Optics, and working on a project way above my pay grade to understand. I knew all that because, since coming out of my coma, I had been receiving a steady stream of emails from him, and among all his lively encouragement – his bloody optimism – I had got a glimpse into his new life. Somewhere, very deep down, I was grateful for his Tigger-ish enthusiasm – and even more so for the long visit he had made to Orlando, supporting my Mum – but at that point in my recovery my outlook on the world could not have been further removed from his. His radiant sunshine found no way through the heavy dark clouds of the low-pressure depression sitting so stubbornly over my life.

Pete had been insisting I head out to Colorado, determined to get me into the fresh air of the mountains ('It's beautiful here! You'll love it!') and to start pushing myself to accelerate my recovery ('It'll do you a power of good, mate! You'll be up those mountains before you know it!'). Politely declining his invitations, I kept telling him I had neither the physical capabilities nor the strength of heart to be beasted by him, or anyone else, in the great American outdoors. I was in very rough shape still. But he never gave up, the bastard, he was like a feisty terrier yanking at my trouser leg. And now he was on the end of the phone, yanking even harder, overruling all my objections with wafting reassurance and cheerfulness. I had kept an ace up my sleeve and thought I had clinched the argument when I finally played it, telling him that I was living off disability benefits and had no money in the bank. But he just brushed that aside. 'To hell with the money – I was hardly expecting you to pay for your own flight, was I? So, how about it? See you here in two weeks?'

Tired of resistance, succumbing to his infuriating charm and superhuman kindness I gave into the inevitable and boarded a goddam flight to Colorado. I was dreading it. Operations for my elbow had been scheduled but my arm was still locked out, the massive hernia was starting to press out of my lower gut, the burn wounds on my head and right shoulder were open, raw and painful, and I was at least two stone overweight from all the meds I had been taking. Tough hiking in the wilderness of the Rocky Mountains was not on my wish list. Pete promised we'd take it easy and besides, he said, he had to work so I'd be just fine, I'd have all day to rest up. Yeah right, Pete.

The last time I had been in an aircraft it had caught fire and I had nearly died, but I wasn't as anxious as I thought I might be when I got airborne again. That was probably because I was too focused on my discomfort. I wasn't used to sitting for such a long period, and especially not in such a confined space. My arm was sticking out into the aisle and my wounds chafed against the seat. But it was more my inner discomfort. I was anxious about the prolonged public exposure. Ducking in and out of the news-agent or Tesco was one thing, but the 15 hours from arriving at Heathrow to being met in Denver was by far the longest time I had spent inflicting my presence on other people.

Three years had passed since I was last out and about like a regular citizen of the world. I had joined my flight-school house-mates for a burger and a beer in a restaurant on the local strip and the only person to look at me twice that evening was the very attractive waitress. If she was on that flight to Denver no doubt she would have looked twice again, but she'd have no clue it was the quite good-looking guy she had flirted with back in August 2007. The great thing about the aircraft cabin, if you were unfortunate enough to have a face like mine, was that we were all facing the same way. The only ones who had to suffer my ugly mug were the cabin crew and, bless them, they were lovely, pretending I was just like anyone else, like I had cut myself shaving maybe. Once I had eaten, I even managed to doze off for a couple of hours.

I hadn't seen Pete for seven years, but he had no trouble recog-nising me at Denver airport. I was the freak, bloated with water retention and hobbling on a walking stick, gasping for breath, my head wrapped in netting and bandages and my face like a grill pan of streaky bacon. He greeted me like I had nothing worse than a head cold. He too was apparently blind to my injuries, and instantly I felt cheered. The only problem was that I could barely speak.

I was gasping for air because of the altitude. Denver is 5,280 feet above sea level – exactly one mile – and even people without health issues struggle to acclimatise to the thin air for a few days. Colorado Springs, where Pete lived, is another thousand feet into the atmosphere. Climbing ever higher in his big redneck's jeep, we wound our way due south on the Interstate 25 highway, the stunning landscape a little lost on me because I was concentrating so hard on getting oxygen in my lungs. Pete had reminded me on the phone that the high mountain air would help my wounds heal, but by the time we reached his lovely home up the hill from the city centre I was really struggling.

I was hoping for a little peace and quiet to help me settle in, but I was immediately disabused of that prospect by Max, Pete's huge and very affectionate dog. Max was a giant of the canine world, more like a cross between a grizzly bear and a shire horse than a Labrador and bullmastiff. You certainly wouldn't want to spill his pint of Pedigree Chum, but as the beast burst from the house, leaped the flowerbed and came bounding down the front yard, Pete assured me that Max was very friendly ... to people he knew. He was certainly very excited to make my acquaintance, leaping up at me, trying to slap his massive paws on my shoulders and lick my face. This was not the treatment recommended by my plastic surgeons in the rehab guidelines, and Pete bellowed at him to get down, eventually having to grab his collar and pull him clear. With my bloody raw wounds, I think he mistook me for a (partially) mobile rump steak. He may not have eaten me but he would no doubt have licked me down to the bone.

Pete went off to work in the mornings and slowly my body grew accustomed to the air. On the third day, I foolishly took up Pete's parting suggestion that I take Max out for 'a short stroll' in the street. It was a decision I regretted the moment I opened the front door and we shot down the path, me virtually horizontal in the air, my good arm clinging on to the dog leash like a cartoon character. I was quite literally dragged up and down the street, and by the time I got back in the house I was panting and drooling, just like Max, and collapsed on the sofa.

For the first week, Pete was as good as his word and he took it easy on me. When his day was done, we'd head into town for a beer or a pizza and go for a short stroll. During the day I rested up and soon I was breathing normally, no longer feeling faint. As soon as I announced that, Pete started pushing me. Quite hard.

Pete being a great organiser, I knew he would have drawn up some sort of fitness schedule for me, and very probably one well beyond what I believed to be the limit of my capabilities. How right I was. On the fifth day of my visit, he started me on a famous local landmark called the Manitou Springs Incline, known to the locals simply as The Incline. Everybody knew The Incline. Some even manage to scale it. The Incline is an arrow-straight trail that heads up a dizzyingly steep slope towards Pike's Peak, the highest summit in the southern Rocky Mountains. It follows the route of a former narrow gauge funicular railway washed away by a rock slide in the 1990s. The prize for walking it is an incredible view, but standing at the foot of it, a photo of it would have suited me just fine. The average gradient is 45 per cent, steep as 68 per cent in places, and you gain over 2,000 feet of elevation in just under a mile.

'You are fucking kidding me, Pete.'

'Come on, Jamie,' he smiled. 'This is nothing for a tough old boot like you.'

I threw him an evil glare and placed a boot on the first of the 2,744 railway sleepers. Over the next week or so, we took a gradual approach to conquering it, each time going that little bit higher until my body screamed in protest and barred me from going any further. On the fifth attempt, I made it to the 2,744th step. Even in the flush of health, I would have been pretty chuffed to have climbed The Incline, so reaching the top in my condition, I now look back on this as one of the greatest feats of endurance I have ever achieved. Seriously, I rank it alongside the Cambrian Patrols, 'P' Company and Selection – perhaps higher. The temperature had been touching 30°C during the day and, although it was the evening, it was still very warm and after a hundred or so steps I was absolutely sodden. And, of course, we were already over a mile up in the atmosphere and the air was thin.

After cardiac arrest, my main worry was falling backwards and cracking my head, breaking a limb or tearing off strips of my delicate paper-thin new skin. The Incline is so steep no car, no matter how light or powerful, could ever get up a gradient that steep. When abseiling or rock-climbing I was always advised never to look down, but on The Incline, you don't want to look up either. Both views induce vertigo. Without shin muscles, balance was a problem for me and even with the walking poles and Pete right behind to catch me, I felt unsteady and anxious all the way up, especially on the severely steep sections. Pete was right there the whole way, as he had been every time, staying quiet for the most part (probably because he didn't have the breath to speak), but urging me on whenever I stopped to refill my lungs and to question whether I was able to make it. At the halfway, his clever response was that it would be far more dangerous and strenuous on the muscles to head back to the foot. On we pushed.

The view is truly something from the top of The Incline but, just a few more railway sleepers from certain death, I was in no state to enjoy it. I sat in the dirt, head down, sweat gushing out of me, lungs heaving and muscles burning. There was zero chance of me making it back down the steps so after half an hour we took the gentle path back to the car, Pete right at my elbow in case I gave out. I was starving from burning off a warehouse of calories but, too tired to eat, I fell into bed and woke up 14 hours later.

Pete was right – after a week I noticed my wounds were clearly healing faster and I was building up some serious fitness. The stubborn misery in me was loath to concede any of its hard-earned ground, but I was rediscovering something vaguely resembling happiness – or what I was able to recall of that state of being. It's not just a figure of speech when I say I had forgotten how to be happy. It had been so long it was hard to recognise the first shoots of it. So it was a strange sensation emerging within me during my time in Colorado – a fresh conflict being waged in my soul, the warring factions being my fury, frustration and fear on the one side and my determination, my appetite for life and hunt for a new happiness – and gratitude to Pete – on the other.

Pete had been was wise to keep his schedule of activities to himself. Had I ever got eyes on the list, I would probably have ordered a cab while he was at work and headed back to Denver airport. I knew he had planned a relaxing road trip for the final week, driving up through Wyoming and east through the Dakotas to Minnesota with his girlfriend (now wife) Janine to stay with her parents at their lakeside holiday home. It was probably just as well he didn't tell me that, before we set off, we were going to climb the notorious Barr Trail, a 13-mile hike up to Pike's Peak. At 14,125 feet, it was a classified as a 'Fourteener' – one of 94 peaks in the United States, all of them west of the Mississippi, the highest 22 of them in Alaska, most of the rest in Colorado. Pike's Peak, ranked 65, was named after soldier and explorer Zebulon Pike in spite of the fact he never made it to the top, he and his men being forced to turn back on their second effort in waist-deep snow.

The Barr Trail is so steep in places that Pete had to 'spot' me, propping me up with an arm or by linking elbows. It's a hike of incredible beauty, the trail winding through pine forests and open meadow in the foothills and emerging gradually into a barren terrain with bizarre rock formations and staggering views. We had set off at 04:30 in the misty grey of pre-dawn but soon there was brilliant sunshine and air so clear you could almost drink it. The climb is just under 8,000 feet from the trailhead and, with every 1,000 feet, the temperature drops three degrees so, in spite of the exertion and it being high summer, we were wearing our cold-weather jackets by the time we reached the higher slopes.

Pete had brought a daysack full of snacks and energy drinks and we both had camel packs, but halfway up we stopped at the coffee shack to rest up before the final push. I was far stronger than when I arrived in Colorado but it's a tough hike for anyone and, much as I was loving it, I was feeling it hard, particularly in my shins. We had gone a few miles up from the shack when I stopped for a pee. Max was off the lead and having the time of his life, bounding in and out of the thinning pines on either side of the trail. But as I was doing up my fly (hard with one working arm!), I heard him erupt in an explosion of barking and growling. Stepping back into the trail, Max had positioned himself about 20 yards in front of us, his muscles tensed in fighting pose, his alarm bark echoing through the woods, foam spilling from his bared teeth.

My first thought was deer, but then the cause of Max's alarm loped out of the trees on to the trail – a huge black bear. It turned and stopped to face us, its dinner-plate paws planted in the dust, eyeing us up, weighing up whether we were worth the effort. There was no more than ten feet between the two animals and Max was doing his utmost to see it off, jumping from side to side, slapping his paws in the dirt and barking like his life depended on it – which it probably did. There was nothing Pete and I could do – we had no gun and I was certainly going to be no use wrestling a bear. I would have struggled with a guinea pig, but with

Max fronting up like that, I wasn't feeling very frightened. That said, I didn't twitch a muscle. The bear never flinched either and, for a minute or so, the scene was suspended in limbo. Looking almost bored and contemptuous, finally the massive carnivore slunk off the trail and into the trees of the descending slope, we thanked Max with some dog biscuits – he was very pleased with himself – and we pushed on.

A few hours later, we made it to the summit, the highest I had ever climbed, and I collapsed like a sack of grain. I was on top of the world in all senses, the view inside me just as spectacular as the one all around. I had the same mixture of pride and exhaustion I used to get in the old days and, thanks to Pete, once I had regained some strength to speak I was able to acknowledge that some of my old confidence was back. My old mate had shown me I still had a life to enjoy and that, with some hard graft and guts, I could recover at least some of what I had lost in the flames. We spent an hour sitting around, taking it all in, gorging ourselves on a picnic, my limbs slowly freezing up, my head fogging with fatigue.

Being an uncertified lunatic, Pete was going to run back down with Max, but I couldn't have crawled another ten yards and he deposited me on to the little tourist train, lifeless as a crate of cargo. From the trailhead, I drove home, showered, fed myself, drove back, sat in the car for an hour, starting to worry a little, when finally, a little head torch came bouncing out of the trees and across the empty car park. Max jumped into the boot and Pete hopped in the front seat, grinning, fresh as a daisy, like he had popped out for some milk.

We spent the final week of my month driving through the spectacular landscapes of the Midwest up to the Great Lakes area near the Canadian border, including a stopover in the Great Sand Dunes National Park, an extraordinary sight among the foothill meadows and the wooded snow-peaked mountains higher up. Americans are the most hospitable people you'll ever meet and Pete's future in-laws are an extreme example of this national characteristic. They could not have been more welcoming. Like everyone else I was meeting, they didn't seem in the least bit disgusted by my bloated, peeling appearance. Lovely people – they treated me like a regular guy and, except when I caught myself in the mirror, I sometimes found myself feeling like a regular guy too, forgetting about my injuries for a while.

As far as you can with Pete, we had a lovely, lazy few days, taking the boat out on to the lake, walking, picnicking and barbequing. It was only right at the end it dawned on me that there had not been one day spent in the company of a nurse or doctor. I have nothing but the greatest admiration for the medical profession, but it was bliss spending some time apart.

I will be forever indebted to Pete Mash for forcibly heaving me out of my gloom, kicking me up the arse and effectively telling me to get on with it. He's far too kind to make a good sergeant major, but he certainly showed all the other attributes to earn his stripes in his brutal but clever and compassionate marshalling of me. Without my mother, I doubt I'd be alive today, but there were many others on the long, hard road of my recovery who kept me going – the men screaming at me in the long grass of the airfield, Renee in Orlando, Pastor Billy at Stoke Mandeville. Pete Mash was another angel to pay me a visit. If the others had brought me back from the brink, Pete gave me the map to find my way back to happiness.

26

On my return to England, I rang the local surgery and booked another appointment with my GP. I had been bothered by so many physical complaints for so long that it was hard to know what to worry about the most. In a way, I was past worrying, the hard worrying at least, but in Colorado, pushing myself to the limit of my physical capabilities, I came to realise that my incisional hernia was more than just an unsightly inconvenience. It was a major problem, and a potentially lethal one, were it to become strangulated. The hernia, a common complication of major abdominal surgery, hung off my waist like I had swallowed a kids' rugby ball. Mine was the legacy of the emergency laparotomy performed in Orlando soon after my accident, the surgeon's last-ditch effort to relieve the bloating caused by the abdominal compartment syndrome and my scorched body's desperate retention of fluids. Focused on the main task of keeping me alive and not wanting to put my body under any greater stress, the surgeons had rightly shied away from stitching me up too tight with sutures or mesh. They never knew when they might have to go back in.

Over time, the abdominis rectus, or my 'six-pack', running from sternum to pelvis bone, had given out to the pressure from the tissue and organs below. Having found a breach in the wall, it came piling through, pushing out further and further. I had become so fat from all the meds that the hernia was lost to some extent among the lumber I was carrying, but walking up all those steps and mountain trails, the hernia bouncing up and down with every stride, I returned home resolved to have the problem addressed as soon as possible. I was sick of the sight of it, sick of the feel of it – and it was a hazard.

Also, it was a truly grotesque appendage and I had quite enough grotesqueness to be getting on with as it was. Again, the physical had an impact on the mental and spiritual. My disfigured and scarred skin made me feel acutely ill-at-ease in public so this great ball of protrusive innards, bouncing over my belt buckle, only deepened my low self-esteem. Thanks to Pete, I was now eager to step up my exercise programme and seek out new challenges and adventures, but all that mountain hiking had proved the hernia was inhibiting basic athletic performance.

I couldn't move on until I got it sorted, but a laparotomy is a serious operation.

Hands in the room don't shoot into the air when surgeons offer a laparotomy. You don't want to have one unless it's crucial to your survival or quality of life. There are big risks, being sliced open like that, most of your vital organs exposed to the elements and infections, and the surgeon's knife always one slip from a disastrous outcome. It's a long operation too and it takes ages to recover – a week or so to start walking and months before you can start taking proper exercise.

There are two schools of thought about how to achieve the best outcome. Some surgeons argue for meshing the stomach wall, others for stitching up the muscle with heavy sutures. It's a tough call because it is not a comparison of like for like. Both methods are meant to be permanent arrangements. With mesh repair there is a smaller chance of the hernia recurring but with the suture there is a lesser likelihood of infection.

My surgeon, Marwan Farouk, opted for mesh repair – and who was I to argue? The operation was performed at High Wycombe

General at the end of July 2010 and Mr Farouk was delighted with his work. True, my hernia had gone; I had a flat stomach again. Who was I to disagree with him? I was delighted to be shot of that mooring buoy of gristle. As it was to turn out, I had every reason to argue with his choice of repair – the quality of his work at least – and every reason to disagree with his cheerful prognosis. More of that later, but for now, I will pause only to tell you that six years later Marwan Farouk was struck off by the General Medical Council for removing a patient's testicle in error, chucking it in the bin on the quiet and failing to inform the man that he was now one ball down. It was a crying shame I didn't have foreknowledge of Mr Farouk's slapdash approach to major surgery.

I was still very much a surgical work-in-progress and in the 18 months following my discharge from Stoke Mandeville I had three more major skin graft operations too. These were all on my right-hand side – the flank which had been blowtorched as I stood on the wing, leaving the deepest burns. The operations on my torso, neck, nose and top lip were performed at Addenbrooke's, Cambridge, by Tariq Ahmad, a consultant plastic surgeon as highly regarded as Dziewulski and Shelley at Chelmsford. Like them, he did an outstanding job, working on the contractures caused by the severe scarring and, once the rawness settled down, I stood before the mirror after every operation and saluted his skills. With each session I was making genuine, visible progress. I was beginning to look almost semi-human and feeling a little sunnier.

It took fully three years, but once my last patch of scorched skin had been grafted, the attention was turned to my lesser problems. My right elbow was the top priority and I underwent three operations to sort it out. I had been very much looking to having my right arm back – my good arm – because, it being stuck fast, I was unable to flex it an inch. All simple daily tasks had to be completed with my left arm and hand – brushing my teeth, eating my food and wiping my arse, ideally in that order. I became almost ambidextrous, a small bonus, I guess, but try using your wrong arm for a few hours and you will soon discover that it is a hugely frustrating inconvenience. Today, I still use my left hand when I need only a fork to eat with, but the development of my new semi-ambidextrous skills stopped short of writing so, before the operations, I was never able to sign my name or dash a quick thank-you to a well-wisher. Unable to put pen to paper, it was probably just as well that typing with the index finger of my left hand was so laborious and tiring. Any quicker and I may have ended up much further down the line with my suicide application to Dignitas.

My elbow operations were performed at High Wycombe by Geoffrey Taylor, a very experienced and charming surgeon of the old-school tradition in whom I had the utmost confidence from the outset. He was frank about the outlook, making it clear I was unlikely to regain full flexibility and could probably lay to rest any dreams I may have entertained about opening the bowling for England or throwing the javelin at the Olympics. He described the procedures as 'a hammer-and-chisel' job, chipping away at the tissue that had calcified and turned into a ball of bone, locking the humerus bone in the upper arm into the ulna in the lower.

With each operation, I was able to bend the arm that much further and by the time he was done, it was as good as new. True, I have never been summoned to team up with the squad at Lord's or roomed with Mo Farah, but I was happy just to be able to touch my face, wash the dishes with both hands, use a knife to cut my food and practise the lost art of handwriting. With every step of physical improvement, there was a corresponding increase in my mood and outlook. Not having someone else chop up my meat, or carve a loaf of bread, did wonders for my self-esteem. I also felt steadier and more confident on my feet. My balance was righted and there was no longer the lingering fear that I might not be able to break my fall if I were to stumble. Confidence, I was constantly being reminded, is built in strange ways.

27

Once my incisional hernia was taken care of – or so it seemed – my focus turned to getting as fit as possible. There was more to my dreams than looking better and feeling good about myself. Colorado had shown me the way out of despair, the way forward. If I could master The Incline and scale a Fourteener, what was to stop me pushing myself even harder? I was going to have to live with my bilateral footdrop for the rest of my days and I was now officially disabled, entitled to all the rights, and condemned to all the stigmas that go with that status. But that wasn't going to stop me testing my capabilities to the max, just like the old days. Sure, I could forget about competitive sport, but that was no problem. I was only ever interested in self-competition – seeing how far I could go, exposing myself to new experiences, the more dangerous the better.

It's weird what upsets you when your whole life, or at least the one you knew and loved, collapses in on itself. I had a very long list of sorrows and disappointments to work through, but high among them was the strong likelihood I would never get to scuba dive again. I just couldn't imagine how that was going to be possible, peeling the tight neoprene suit on to and off my delicate skin, the saltwater, the beating sun, the heavy air tank on my back, the straps digging into my shoulders, the weight belt constricting my waist, the airtight mask sucking my face and the hard rubber fins biting into my feet.

Diving had been my one great passion for over 12 years. It was my escape and refuge, my retreat into another world, away from all the worries and stresses above the surface. It was my regular hit of adrenaline too. I liked to dive deep and I liked to dive the tough locations. I had qualified as a Master Instructor – the highest rating – with the Professional Association of Diving Instructors, the biggest and best dive organisation in the world, and my PADI certificate was also my passport to exotic lands. I had taken my diving gear all over the world and, thanks to the diving community, I had made incredible, unlikely friends from all cultures and backgrounds.

I was going to miss diving like I was going to miss a limb, but the way to deal with that painful loss in my life was obvious: I had to replace it with other activities, get my thrills and experiences from elsewhere. Combining this urgency for a new challenge with the need to get fit, I set my mind on running the 2011 London Marathon the following April. Or rather, walking the London Marathon, because running, except over very short distances, was still very much in the planning stage. That gave me about six months to get into some kind of shape, and it gave me a focus to my day and a structure to my weeks.

At the start of October 2010, two months after the laparotomy, my stomach muscles were strong enough to put them under stress without fear of my innards forcing their way out again. I headed back into the Dunstable Downs to start a strict walking programme, increasing the distance I covered at the start of each week. By January I was doing a 12-mile walk every other day and I would continue to do that until I set off on the big race from Greenwich Park on 17 April 2011.

* * *

What I liked most about the 2011 London Marathon was getting lost in the crowd. It was the most sustained and glaring public appearance I had made since my accident. There were even television cameras beaming the pictures into millions of homes. Of course, no one gave a flying toss about me, but that's to miss the point about acute self-consciousness. It was inspiring too to see many runners with disabilities and injuries far graver than mine, including veterans running on prosthetics or wheeling themselves in chairs. I walked it with an ex-army mate, Rob, who I knew to be a keen runner and I had contacted to see if he could help get me a starting place. (You don't just rock up for the marathon; it's hard to get on to it.) Rob introduced me to his friend (soon to be mine) Des Stockdale, a no-nonsense London businessman, who arranged our gold bond charity places in the line-up. Rob was running to raise money for Keech Hospice in Luton, where Des's late mother had received incredible care. I joined him in the cause and we succeeded in raising about £6,000, specifically for the hospice's terminally ill children's ward.

It was a blazing hot day and it was probably just as well I was walking the marathon because I would have struggled even if I had been fully able-bodied. It was an achievement to cross the line – in eight hours, twenty minutes. Over six hours after the Kenyan winner of the men's race, but who cares who wins? It's who dares wins. I dared to take part. I cared only that I was having a great day out in the sun with a bunch of loons in fancy dress being cheered all the way by tens of thousands of spectators. It was very difficult not to enter into the spirit of fun when you spend over eight hours in the company of a man dressed in an old-fashioned diving suit complete with heavy bell helmet.

As my scalp and shoulder were still pretty tender, the skin not fully knitted yet, I wore bandages to keep off the beating sun and by the time we crossed the line in Hyde Park the dressings were sodden with sweat. Deliberately I hadn't walked further than 12 miles during my training, but I never doubted I'd complete the 26 miles. I had bought an excellent pair of trainers and I knew from my army days how to 'admin' myself well, taking on plenty of fluids and energy snacks and pacing myself evenly. It was tough and I was hanging on by the end, Rob keeping up my morale when I hit the wall around the 18-mile mark. I had been used to crossing lines first not last but, collapsing into a foil heat blanket, I felt as though I had won. It was probably just as well that Rob and I were staying at the Special Forces Club, a stone's throw from the finish line, because I am not sure I could have made it any further.

Inspired by the experience, the following week I applied to run the New York Marathon, the most oversubscribed of all the marathons. I love the States and I had always wanted to spend some time in New York. The race was on 6 November so once I had let my body recover from London, I resumed my regular walks up in the Dunstable Downs and, for a change of scenery, the gentle beauty of the Chiltern Hills. This time I turned to my old cockney mate Andy Coleman to help get a place in the line-up. Andy is a fitness trainer and a top-class long-distance runner who once came second in the Great North Run and, exploiting his contacts in the world of athletics, he was able to secure me a starting place.

Staying in a fancy apartment just few hundred yards from the finishing line in Central Park made the experience even more memorable. It belonged to the son of a woman Andy trained in London and we were very fortunate and grateful to have such a convenient and luxurious base with its incredible views of the skyline from the fifteenth floor. It was like being in a film set, a stream of honking yellow cabs down on the street and a guy under the entrance awning greeting us each time we came or went with a touch of his top hat.

We were just about to head into the elevator to head off to the race when I received a text with the sad news that my gran, my father's mum, had finally passed away after a long struggle. I was pleased she had been released from her suffering, but I loved her very much – she looked after me a lot when I was very young – and I was feeling pretty choked up in the melee behind the starting line. Her death added to the emotion of a highly charged day. I had loved the London Marathon, but this atmosphere was something else. What is it about Americans and their enthusiasm? From the moment I crossed the bridge from Staten Island into Brooklyn, dozens of helicopters buzzing overhead, I was carried along by a truly extraordinary tide of energy and goodwill from fellow runners and spectating New Yorkers.

I had been given a pink tank-top with my name and the number 151 on front and back and, no kidding, for almost the entire race people were cheering me on: 'Go, Jamie, Go! ... Go for it, Pink 151! ... You're going to do it, Jamie! ... You can do this, man!' About halfway, I emerged from a railway tunnel and was met by a big sign saying *Welcome to Queens* and a guy in a reverse baseball cap with a big grin and a reefer in his hand jumping up and down shouting, 'Hey dude, yeah, as it says, welcome to Queens but if you don't want to stay here we understand. You push on, man. We'll be just fine!'

Crossing the Queensboro Bridge and Roosevelt Island, the course heads on to Manhattan and up to the Bronx before turning south for the final five miles to Central Park. It was all amazing but the Bronx was the liveliest area, the streets pulsing with heavy beats from speakers in windows and on the steps up to the houses. There were two guys with their own amp and microphones banging out some heavy rap and, as I went by, they punched the air and sang, 'You can do it! You can do it!'

Being that bit stronger, I had decided to powerwalk most of the course, which is a much heavier effort than plain walking but, the rappers were right, I knew I could do it. Andy had long disappeared to run the race properly and he would have been finished for hours by the time I launched my push on the final few miles. The light was dropping and I could see my breath in the cold November air, but I had fallen in with a bunch of very friendly US veterans, a lot of them blade-running amputees, and we chatted and encouraged each other right to the end. I was very close to tears when I crossed the line. London had been a buzz, but New York was emotional. Perhaps it was linked to my feelings of grief, but there was not one step of the way when I didn't feel the heavy electric charge of the atmosphere, a powerful sense of connection with my fellow man. For the record, I crossed the line in seven hours and seven minutes. I was getting physically stronger too.

28

With the physical area of my life back up and running again – or walking, rather – I turned my attention to the next great challenge, one that was going to take all my moral and mental strength, the outcome of which was going to have a major bearing on the rest of my life: the legal fight for compensation. I had spent seven years working towards selection in one of the most revered military units in the world and, having just reached my goal, that opportunity was torn away from me through no fault of my own. I was a young man, and a man of action, with a long working life ahead of me. I had suffered three years of sheer hell, I had lost my looks, my mobility, my confidence, most of my pastimes, my romantic life and probably my chances of becoming a husband and a father. I had years of plastic surgery ahead of me, years of physical pain and discomfort and mental anguish. I had lost my hopes and dreams. How do you put a price on that?

I was about to find out. I called my American lawyer Joe and instructed him to start preparing my case.

In the seven months between the two marathons I made two trips to Orlando to see my lawyers. I had high hopes of a generous settlement for the devastation of my life caused by someone else's negligence or recklessness, but the stress of the coming battle had been eating at my guts. I was up against the chicanery of the US legal system and the power of unseen institutional forces dictating the outcome.

I liked Joe. Dressed in a sharp grey suit, he met me off the plane on my first visit and checked me into the hotel right there above the terminal concourse at Orlando International. He spoke openly and frankly, full of optimism but cautious about the mighty obstacles that lay before us. When I boarded my BA flight to Heathrow, I was happy I had the right man on my side and full of hope that justice was going to be done. I fell into a deep sleep, pleased at the thought that, whatever else lay in store for me, at least money wasn't going to be a worry.

When I went back to Orlando at the end of the summer, as we pulled off the airport access road on to the 436 beltway Joe told me we would be up against a team of heavy-hitters with the full power of the aviation industry behind them. He confessed he was starting to feel a little outgunned, so wanted to call in some artillery of his own in the form of a specialist in aviation law.

Joe's office was a reassuringly modest affair set in a strip of nondescript buildings on a run-of-the-mill stretch of street. He was a one-man band, a young PA called Britney his only colleague, and the office was quiet. I liked that. I was sitting by the window, the strong sun beating on the window and the air conditioner going full tilt, when our aviation expert made his entrance.

A spotless red Corvette pulled into the half-empty parking lot out front, the door opened and out swung a pair of gleaming cowboy boots. The massive guy who stood up in them placed a huge cowboy hat on his head and yanked the belt on his chinos up over his considerable gut. Don was quite a character. Tossing his cowboy hat on to the table, he greeted me with a firm hand-shake and a beaming smile.

'It's a great pleasure and real honour meeting you, Jamie. Mind if I call you, Jamie? I am so sorry to hear about your accident and I am in awe of you for making it through. I'm going to be fighting tooth and nail for you.'

Don and I sat down and I told him the story of my accident minute by minute and, when it came to the fire and the crash, second by second. He had been a military helicopter pilot before training as a lawyer and it was greatly reassuring that he knew about flying and the mechanics of aircraft.

Don was soon in a state of high excitement about the case. 'This is incredible, Jamie! Incredible. Real excited about representing you on this.'

I liked Don, but I didn't know whether I was right to trust in his enthusiasm. In a way it was reassuring when he added, 'But we mustn't get our hopes too high at this stage. One important thing I learned in the military was never underestimate your enemy, Jamie. Never.'

I nodded and we watched Don pull on to the street with a guttural roar from the Corvette's exhausts.

I turned to Joe. 'What wars did Don fight in?'

'Er, none, as far as I know.'

• • •

Colorado, Orlando twice, New York – in 2011, I was spending almost as much time in the States as I was in the UK and towards the end of the year I was given yet another opportunity to visit.

I had received so much support and goodwill over the previous four years that, as I recovered, I began to feel a growing urgency to reverse the flow of kindness and start helping others. This wasn't just a question of conscience. It was an emotional rather than a moral calling. Pathetically dependent on the goodness of others for so long, I had come to understand the true meaning of suffering and I felt irresistibly compelled to help out others experiencing similar pain and torment in any which I was capable. The obvious and quickest way to 'put something back' was through an organisation with the infrastructure, the know-how and the opportunities already in place. So, in the latter half of 2011, I became involved with two military charities, Pilgrim Bandits and Help for Heroes.

Pilgrim Bandits is a small, punchy charity established by Special Forces veterans in 2007 to help and inspire wounded soldiers to live life to the full, by pushing them beyond what they believed were the limits of their capabilities – climbing mountains, white-water kayaking, hiking through inhospitable terrain, skydiving, anything that involves endurance or buckets of adrenaline. My task was to help fly the flag for them, raising money and their profile. They do a great deal of work with ex-paratrooper Ben Parkinson. I soon got to know him well and we have remained close friends. Ben is a very cool dude who wears a very brave and smiling face in spite of suffering just about the worst set of injuries imaginable, sustained when his vehicle drove over a 20-year-old Russian anti-tank mine in Afghanistan in 2006. The blast broke his back in three places, shattered every rib, punctured his lungs, ruptured his spleen and smashed up his jaw. He sustained 35 distinct injuries in all, both his legs were amputated above the knee and he was left with debilitating brain damage that stole his power of speech.

His cheerful personality radiates through the suffering and he has been a great inspiration to me as I battled my own problems, spending a lot of time with him up at his parents' house in Doncaster and at various fundraising events. He's one of those people who, no matter how you're feeling, puts you in a good mood the moment you enter his company. Thanks to his own efforts, plus the support of Pilgrim Bandits and some pioneering new treatments, it gives me genuine delight each time I hear from him or from his mother Diane that he has made even more progress in his recovery.

At around the same time that I became involved with Pilgrim Bandits, I was contacted by Help for Heroes and invited to join their Band of Brothers network – a mutual support group for wounded ex-servicemen. The arrangement works on a give-and-take basis – they help you and you help them in any which way you can. At first, I was taking more than giving but I soon became heavily involved in representing and furthering their cause, participating in dozens of events in their name. I got a call from them not long after my return from the New York Marathon, asking if I would like to take part in a trip to Utah the week before Christmas and learn to become a pilot.

'A pilot! Thank you but I don't think so,' I laughed nervously down the phone. 'My last effort at qualifying as a pilot hadn't turned out so well.'

'No, we mean a bobsleigh pilot! To be trained by the US Olympic team.'

I needed no further urging. Since recovering some mobility and some morale, my appetite for activities had become ravenous. After years moping in a bed, I wanted to gorge myself on as much life as I could cram in.

'Go on, twist my rubber arm. When do we leave?'

I flew out to Salt Lake City in mid-December 2011 as part of an eight-strong British team to train and compete alongside veterans from Wounded Warrior and Soldier On, respectively the US and Canada counterparts of our Help for Heroes. Each unit had its own support staff, volunteers from the charities, and we were trained as two-man teams on the bobsleigh runs used in the 2002 Winter Olympics.

I was hungry for thrills, but I began to have second thoughts about volunteering when the instructors took us to the head of the course and we looked down the steep, twisting tracks. Once you're on a bobsleigh there's no getting off and it's impossible to stop. It's a terrifying and dangerous sport and we all looked at each other, cracking nervous jokes. But with Olympic-standard coaches running the show, we were in extremely capable hands and they gave us little time to dwell on the fearful consequences of screwing it up. They took us back down and started us out on the lowest stretch of track, taking us higher and higher over the course of the week, the instructors, not the competitors, deciding if we had achieved sufficient proficiency to move up to the next level. It was a thrill just to be in this stunning landscape of the snow-plastered Rockies, with bright blue skies every day.

I started off as a brake man at the rear with an instructor steering in the front, but soon we were doing it as proper teams, our efforts recorded on video to assess the margins of our errors. I hadn't experienced such a happy rush of adrenaline since learning to fly in Florida and I found the sensation and the danger utterly exhilarating from the off. The higher you go, the faster you descend. I was determined to make it to the starting line at the top from where you hit speeds touching 80mph.

It was one of the best weeks of my life – not just since my accident – and that was partly because the Americans, the Canadians and our instructors were brilliant company. At the end of each exhausting, nerve-jangling day, we hit the bars and, buzzing for hours, we gabbled and bantered over rounds of beers. Never much of a drinker, I had become physically incapable of having more than two or three pints, but it didn't stop me having a blast with the others. If Pete Mash had shown me the route to happiness, these guys showed me how to laugh again. The wounded veteran charities are magnificent if only for laying on these shared experiences for people who had come to believe that fun was just something people enjoyed.

On the last day, I was considered good enough to make the full run and I was bricking it as I wriggled down at the front of the sled. As most of the guys had leg injuries, there was no running start – the instructors just gave us a nudge and a way we flew. This is how it must feel to fly an aircraft in an open cockpit. You are accelerating for the first 90 per cent of the track, the G-force becoming ever more powerful. Concentrating so hard on not making a mistake and flipping the sled, there is no time or head space to feel frightened. By the time we reached the upward slope at the foot and my teammate yanked on the brake lever, I was laughing and shaking with sheer joy.

It had been some time since I had felt quite so happy to be alive – alive! – and I boarded the plane home just before Christmas, pumped by the possibilities that lay ahead. I didn't have to wait long for my next heart-jacking experience. I had barely walked in the door and said hello to my mum when my mobile rang. Help for Heroes was wondering if I would like to go back to North America for a winter sports activity camp in Vancouver – the whole trip funded by the charity. Does the Pope kiss tarmac? Do bears powder their noses in the woods? Just over a week later, on New Year's Day 2012, I was back at Heathrow.

The activities were different but the landscape, the company, the challenge, the thrills, the sense of achievement and the camaraderie were identical to those I had experienced in Salt Lake City. Again, the Brits joined teams of Americans and Canadians and again we all got on like long-lost brothers at a surprise reunion party. Most of the veterans had lost a limb in combat, but the way it was organised and supervised, being an arm or leg down was not going to stop any one of us from Nordic skiing, competing in biathlons and ice-sledge hockey, dogsledding and racing skidoos through the wooded mountains. Two of the US vets had suffered severe burns and I bonded particularly strongly with them, sharing our experiences and welcoming the comforting knowledge that we had all been through the same appalling ordeal. There was good deal of mickey-taking between the units of the respective militaries and some very un-PC jokes and barbs about our disabilities. To an outsider, this may have sounded shocking, but for us it was a wonderful release to make light of our conditions through the soldier's favourite form of communication – banter.

North America may have been the scene of the great misfortune in my life, but it was now turning out to be my salvation. America was rebuilding me, physically and spiritually. I was becoming addicted to the beauty of the landscape and the energy of its people. This was probably why, not long after my return, I made possibly the craziest decision of my life – to compete in the Race Across America, the world's toughest bicycle race. The event was to take place in June 2012, starting near San Diego on the Californian coast down by the Mexican border. You cover 3,000 miles and, racing non-stop, day and night, the hope is you reach Annapolis, Maryland, on the eastern seaboard about a week later.

I had lost a great deal in the flames of my burning aircraft, but my friends were now openly wondering whether my sanity had gone up in smoke too.

29

I went into training the day after I got back. Apart from a few short workouts with the physios in Stoke Mandeville on an exercise bike, I hadn't cycled in earnest for over five years and I was puffing after just a mile along the flat roads near my home. The main muscles we use for cycling are different to those needed for running and walking and I had read somewhere that multiple Tour de France winner Miguel Induráin feels the strain of walking upstairs even when he is at peak cycling fitness. That sounded ridiculous to me – but now I got it.

Foolishly perhaps, I had also signed up for another London Marathon in April 2012 – my third 26-miler in 12 months. My mania for activity, suspended for so many years, had now gone into overdrive and I was worried I may have taken on too much. With the charity work, my legal fight and regular visits to doctors and surgeons, my daily schedule, so empty so recently, was starting to fill to overflowing.

These big-city marathons are great for the soul as much as the body and it was worth it, this third time out, just for feeding off the buzzing energy and goodwill of the cheering spectators. There was not the enormous sense of achievement I had felt in my first race, but I pushed myself hard, jogging the occasional stretch, the bilateral footdrop making me a look like a duck in a hurry to find his haemorrhoid cream. I crossed the line with a pack of other stragglers in a respectable six hours and fifteen minutes and, this time, there was still some crowd left over the closing miles to help me stagger to the finish.

By then, I had made the selection cut for the Race Across America (RAAM). For months, I had joined about 20 hopefuls every weekend at Tedworth House in Wiltshire, Help for Heroes' recovery centre in the south, to prove we might be able to last the distance. RAAM is a non-stop team effort, the cyclists in each team sleeping and riding in relays. The only time you stop is when the pairs change over, two emerging from the back of the touring vans and two heading in for some chow and sleep. I was enjoying the experience of working in a team again, just as I had in Salt Lake City and in Vancouver – and in my time with the military. More than ever, the sense of belonging to a group with a shared goal gave me a deep satisfaction. In true *esprit de corps*, there were no hard feelings among those who failed to make the final eight.

Not long after the marathon, I boarded a flight to Orlando, my third visit since my accident, to make my deposition, the formal and final written statement of the events giving rise to my legal case and quest for damages. Joe drove me around again while I was there and on my second day, I asked if he could take me to Orlando Regional Medical Center, so that I could meet the staff in the Burns Unit of the Trauma Center. Joe readily agreed. He knew as well as anyone what that Burns Unit meant to me.

I was very excited to go back – and yet, in a way, I was going there for the first time. I had no idea what it looked like. But I owed the staff there my life. They had worked wonders. I am going to be forever grateful for the incredible care they gave me. Perhaps all emergency healthcare in the States is the same but I find it hard to believe that, had I been taken anywhere else but Orlando, I would have made it through. Much of that conviction derives from what I had been told about my lead nurse, Renee. When I arrived on the helipad, a dead man screaming, some of the admissions team had no hope I'd make it and believed any effort expended on me was futile. They felt the humane route, quietly letting me go, was the kindest and most credible option – knock me out with drugs and let nature takes its inevitable course. But Renee was the most vocal in fighting the case for life, insisting I was given the best possible chance. That's what Mum says and I have no reason to doubt her.

What is also not in doubt is that Renee was right at my side, battling for me, during those first critical weeks and months. I have no conscious memory of her, no visual images, but I can still hear her voice today, feel her presence, the power of her spirit. I am not a goggle-eyed mystic, or even especially religious in a conventional sense, but I believe that my connection with her through the deep coma kept me alive. I think I was slightly in love with her. I think I still am. I was excited and nervous in equal measure finally to make her acquaintance.

The reception desk called up to the ward and about five minutes later an orderly appeared to escort us up. We headed into the elevator for the third floor, and my heart was going some. We put on our scrubs and I squelched down the corridor in my rubber shoes, looking around, taking in the details and soaking in the atmosphere of the place that had been my home for three months. It was a weird sensation to visit somewhere I had lived for so long and yet had not the merest recollection of it – other than that lovely, ghostly girl's voice.

Word that I was down at reception had gone out and by the time I reached the nurses' station, opposite my old room, nurses and doctors were appearing from everywhere. Soon, there was a gathering of about 30, a big smile wrapping every face. Of course, I didn't recognise a single face but most of these people knew me more intimately than I could ever truly understand. They had cut me open, massaged and probed my vital organs, stitched me up, patched me up with dead men's skin, cleaned and dressed my wounds, washed me, wheeled me, changed my sheets, worked my limbs, emptied bags of my piss and my crap, smeared me in ointments, gave me food, fluids and medication, talked to me, bigged me up, monitored my vital signs, maybe even said prayers for me.

This posse of grinning strangers had nursed me back from the very brink of death – time and time again – and I was so overwhelmed I was barely able to speak. There was a carnival of handshaking, hugging and smiling, the air full of congratulations and thanks and mutual awe. It was a wonderful moment for me, but afterwards I realised it must have been quite something for them too. I was a dramatic example of what made their work worth all that massive and stressful effort, a living, walking, talking demonstration of why, occasionally, they get to love their jobs in a way denied to almost every other professional.

Reviving a dehydrated houseplant is the closest most of us get to the miracle of restoring life to a dying organism. When the casevac helicopter delivered me to them, I looked like an overdone hog roast, blood and fluids seeping through the charred crust. I was given about a 5 per cent chance of survival. Now, thanks to them, here I was, three-and-a-half years later, walking (almost normally) in jeans, shirt and baseball cap, shaking hands, embracing, talking and joking. I had never said a word when I was here – except very occasionally when I garbled like a sleep-talker – and now, overcoming my nerves, I could barely shut my mouth. I made a little speech – not my best but I think the emotion and gratitude found a way through the nerves. They gave me a big clap, and there were quite a few tears wiped away.

Everyone came to greet me individually afterwards and when the group started to break up and they headed back to their work, I carried on scanning the faces for Renee. Thinking about it later, I knew in my guts that she wasn't there. I think I would have recognised her instantly just by the way she would have been looking at me. There would have been a connection. As I was about to leave, I asked one of the senior nurses if she could point out Renee, explaining that I wanted to offer special thanks to her for all that she had done for me as my lead clinician. A shadow fell over the nurse's face and she looked at the floor. She exhaled hard, put a hand on my shoulder, and said,

'Renee died about a year ago. I'm sorry, Jamie.'

I stared at her for a few moments, my mouth drying. 'How?'

'Terrible accident on the freeway. It was instant. She didn't suffer. I'm so sorry. We knew you'd really want to see her.'

She held on to my shoulder for a while longer, then drew me in and gave me a hug.

'Jamie, I have to get back to work, but it's a joy to see you looking so great and, yes, I'm so, so sorry. We all are. It was a huge shock. We miss her.'

For a few moments I didn't move, and the others let me be. I looked up, through the glass door into Room Ten. A body lay in the bed, bound in bandages from head to knee, his face covered with a sort of jellied mask, a dozen cables and tubes hanging out of him hooked up to banks of equipment and bags of fluids. I shook some more hands, hugged some more bodies and headed out slowly, Joe placing a friendly arm on my shoulder.

30

The next day we headed out to the airfield and the scene of my accident. Joe had told me a year back that the flight school had grounded the planes that were the same model I'd flown in, after a second serious accident. But there was still plenty of activity around the hangars on my return. We sat in the car and watched a couple of light aircraft landing and taking off, the squat control tower in the distance, close to where I had bailed out and the plane had exploded.

At the deposition meeting later that day, we were up against the flight school, the plane's manufacturers and the company responsible for the maintenance of the aircraft. I had felt such a burning sense of injustice every conscious day since the accident, I had naively convinced myself that the lawyers would accept the version of events as they had happened, hand me a wedge of cash and I could fly home and try and get on with my life. So, I was taken aback, angered even, by the line of questioning, the aim of which was to undermine confidence in my account of what had happened in the cockpit.

Through no fault of his own, Joe had been unable to find one witness to make a statement that they had seen the aircraft coming in on fire. Just one dog walker or one golfer, and that would have made their case impossible to defend. The drama had unfolded very quickly and it was probably only when I was very low, the last 10 or 15 seconds, when a passer-by in the far distance might just have spotted the tiny, stricken plane. But it was a very large airfield in a sleepy area, surrounded by woodland, and it being an airfield, there were no residential homes or streets close by with a view of the runways.

Joe initially hadn't been too worried about the lack of witnesses off the street because there were always the two guys in the control tower. It had been a shock to be told by Joe that his attempts to speak to the controllers on duty that day had run into a solid wall of silence and that, when he had turned up at the airfield in person, he had been shown the hand and repeatedly given the words *No Comment*. I was astonished that the controllers could not be compelled to give sworn evidence, especially in the case of an accident with such catastrophic consequences as mine.

In spite of the deafening silence of these crucial witnesses, we remained hopeful of a good outcome in the final settlement. The nature of the accident and the nature of my injuries spoke for themselves and proved a version of events that was obvious even to a child of four. And we had the photographs of the crash scene to prove them. An Irish flight student living with me in the airfield's courtesy house had rushed to the scene of the crash and, flames still roaring, he had taken loads of pictures. Submitted as evidence, you did not need to be an air accident investigator to work out that not even the Terminator could have crawled out of that inferno and wreckage.

One of their lawyers stood out from the glazed faces, highly impressive and articulate when he spoke and, from his sympathetic facial gestures, a good guy to boot. Out on the driveway, everyone getting into their flash cars, he came over to speak to Joe and me. 'That's one hell of an account, Jamie. I salute you. You have shown remarkable strength of character.'

He was laying on the kindness quite thick, and it seemed genuine and heartfelt. I don't know whether Joe was just entering into the spirit of awe and admiration, or he sensed an opportunity to ram home the suffering I had been through, but he turned to me and said, 'Jamie, if you're not embarrassed, why don't you show him your torso?'

I peeled off my shirt and they both sucked in their breath. The lawyer took a step backwards, muttering 'Oh my God! Oh my God! Boy, you have really been through it, haven't you?'

Joe said to him, 'I'm glad you get it. You see what he's had to endure. Through no fault of his own. That's why we want a fair settlement.'

I boarded my flight still full of hope that I was soon to receive my rightful compensation for the destruction caused to my life. But I took my aisle seat with a touch of paranoia gnawing at my mind that a deal had already been done behind my back and that we were just going through the motions.

As I dozed into an edgy sleep, my thoughts drifting from lawyers and back to Renee. With the legal matters to contend with, I hadn't had the time to take on board the shocking news of her death. As the plane lifted off the runway I was starting to feel pretty choked up about this mystery woman who had done so much to keep me alive and now, in a grim irony, she herself was dead. The flight attendant reached me with her trolley, beaming from side to side with a mouthful of sparkling perfect teeth. But the smile vanished when she looked down at me.

'Are you all right you, sir? Are you in pain? You look—'

'It's okay,' I said. 'Just a bit of hay fever.'

• • •

I would have loved to have gone to court, no matter what the outcome. I would have had my say, spelling out in plain language the truth of my experience for everyone to hear. But I had neither the financial backing, the will, the time nor the strength to spend however many more years stuck in the US justice system, and at God knows what expense. After losing so much of my life – the prime of my life – I desperately wanted to get on with it again as best I could.

My body wasn't fully fixed either. I had years of skin procedures ahead of me, I had and still have problems with my heart, my hearing, my eyesight, my digestion and, of course, my legs and feet. My biggest worry, though, was just starting. Nine months after my second laparotomy, I had started to feel some discomfort and bloating in my lower abdomen. Quite literally, I felt in the pit of my guts that something was amiss. Then there was the urgency of getting by day to day, financially. Still living off state support, I had virtually no money in my bank account. I needed money to rebuild my life, no matter how negligible. I was cornered and the lawyers knew it.

So, taking my lawyers' advice that going to a court was a risk and I could end up with nothing, the case was to be settled through mediation. I wasn't happy with the deal that was offered, as I would have to admit liability in order to get any compensation at all. It would be there on the record that it was my errors, my inexperience, Jamie Hull the bloody fool, who had caused the accident. That would hurt more than the pain of receiving a tiny fraction of my true entitlement. The law is truly an ass: I would be made liable for it all, and yet I would be given a lump sum of compensation by the people who claim it was my fault.

But Don, the cowboy-hat-wearing aviation expert, said to me, 'We are not prepared to go to court with this. Either you sign on the dotted line or we walk away and you find yourself new lawyers.'

'Fuck it. I'll sign,' I said.

Out in the driveway, we all quickly shook hands, everyone desperate to get away, me included. Don gave me a slap on the back, fired up another cigar and climbed into his Corvette. Joe drove me back to the airport, stopping for some ribs and beer and a post-mortem. I asked Joe to be honest about how he felt about the deal. He made no attempt to bullshit me with lawyer smooth talk.

'Very disappointed. For you, not me.'

He meant it. I thanked him for doing his best for me and we went our ways on good terms. I'll always like him.

A sad addendum to the proceedings was that, a couple of weeks later, Joe called to tell me that Don and his wife were on holiday in the Bahamas when he suffered a cardiac arrest and died.

31

I was glad that my legal fight had been settled before I turned up on the starting line of the Race Across America under the 2,000-foot-long wooden pier at Ocean Beach, California, on 16 June 2012. Blood coursing with stress-induced cortisol if the case had remained unresolved, I would probably have suffered a heart attack somewhere along the 3,000-mile coast-to-coast bike route. The race was quite challenging enough – and then some – without that extra heavy load of pressure. Without being conscious of it, I am sure that my decision to settle the case was, in small part, influenced by the fact I was competing in this incredibly tough endurance race, the world's most gruelling, the organisers claim.

Open to amateurs and pros, solo riders and teams of two, four and eight, RAAM – twice the length of the Tour de France – is rightly regarded as one of the great challenges in world sport, even more so if you happen to be shy of a limb or two, as many competitors are. You have to reach the finishing line in the famous old sailing town of Annapolis in under nine days, but the winners would be there in five and most of the others in about seven-and-a-half. It was a daunting thought that over the week ahead, we would climb over 175,000 feet – about six Mount Everests – cross 12 states, three major mountain ranges (Sierra, Rockies and Appalachians), four famous rivers (Colorado, Mississippi, Missouri and Ohio), two deserts (Sonoran and Mojave) and the seemingly endless, windswept expanse of the Great Plains. It had always been a dream to take some time to cross that great country, but I could never have imagined I'd be doing it in a week, and on a pedal bike. It was unlikely I'd see much of it, however. Either I was going to be head down, eyes on the asphalt, legs pumping, or it would be dark. I wanted to take much of the night cycling in order to avoid exposing my sensitive new skin to the elements, particularly so in the intense heat of the deserts. When I wasn't in the saddle, I'd be trying to grab a few hours' sleep in the back of the Winnebago.

Known collectively as Team Battle Back, our British contingent was split into two teams of four – Alpha and Bravo – with each containing a pair of us on road bikes and a pair of hand cyclists on recumbents. Most riders take on the RAAM challenge to raise money and we were representing Help for Heroes, on course to bring in a whopping £100,000 if we could do it within the nine days.

All of us were veterans who had been badly wounded one way or another and there were just seven legs between the eight of us – and the two I brought to the party had a pair of partially paralysed feet attached to them. I was to share the road cycling in Alpha with my RAAM race buddy, ex-Parachute Regiment soldier Rab Smedley, who had suffered a broken neck and spine in a high-speed army skiing accident. The other two upright cyclists, in Bravo, were Sergeant Mark Allen who had lost a leg in a parachute accident, and Royal Marine Don McLean, who suffered damage to his feet when he stepped on an IED.

The four recumbent cyclists had more Steves than legs between them. There was Private Steve Richardson, Staff Sergeant Steve Arnold, Royal Marine Commando Joe Townsend and Sergeant Simon Harmer. They had all lost legs in the Afghanistan campaign. Apart from Mark Allen, who I knew a little, we were all strangers thrown together by this gruelling challenge, but the bonding that had begun during training back at Tedworth

House was soon forged into firm friendships in the furnace of the deserts and the gut-wrenching grind up the mountains. They were a fabulous bunch of guys and it was an honour I'll never forget to ride with them.

It was such a massive operation that we needed a support group of 17, working almost as hard as us, only from the comfort of our Winnebago homes, maintenance vans and the race control wagon at the rear. It was a perpetual relay and while one team was out on the road, the others would be in the van getting rest and replenishments, racing ahead to the next rendezvous point for the handover. It worked the same within each team. If the handover team took place at night, for safety reasons, as the waiting cyclist, ferried forward in a van, you would be stationary at the side of the road, ready to go when your partner came in. He went ahead a little and you overtook him – that way you could be sure that the team had covered every yard across the country. During the day, as the next cyclist you would already be on the move when your partner came level with your back wheel and away you'd go. Each team alternated between its upright cyclists and its two recumbents, so if you were on flat terrain, the two hand cyclists would do about four hours each, then switch to the uprights who each would do the same time in the saddle. On and on it went like this, through state after state, every transition a mad rush and moment of high tension.

The first half of the race, looking at the map, appeared to be the toughest, with two deserts and two mountain ranges to negotiate. In mid-June, the mercury can hit 40°C in the Mojave and Sonoran deserts, and although you get a bit of cool from the breeze you're generating, the sweat drying as fast as it pours, you are losing water like a burst mains pipe. We drank litres and litres of water and energy drinks as we pedalled, never once feeling the need to go for a slash.

We were so focused, the effort so intense, that the incredible landscape shot by and the memories were lost in a blur. I can remember the race region by region, by its terrain, but no more specifically than that. I do vividly remember the giant paddling pool the organisers had laid on as the race headed out of the desert. We had a two-hour wait for the handover from Team Bravo and we jumped into that water like, well, kids into a paddling pool, wallowing and resting our aching limbs, our eyes trying not to wander to the jagged outline of the Rockies on the horizon.

It's probably a mistake before the race to examine the graph profile of the heights of the stages awaiting competitors. The first 1,200 miles, we knew, was all steepling peaks and the rest pretty flat before we would reach the much smaller peaks of the Appalachians towards the end. But these graphs are deceptive because some of the highest peaks may be a gentler, longer climb up switchbacks, while some of the smaller ones might be a short, sharp, steep straight up the slope. We had all begun to look at the lovely flatlining of the graph representing the route across the Great Plains but, in the event, it was on the level that we pulled some of the hardest cycling – and our team got landed with an especially tough shift.

The tornado country of Kansas may be flat as the proverbial pancake but, my God, when the wind got up, I was dreaming of mountains and deserts again. The state is over 400 miles wide and Alpha covered half of it overnight, battling into winds of 50mph, clouds of crop dust swirling around the bike, the grit getting into the mouth and the eyes. The wind was so strong, at times, I was barely moving forward, the effort as strenuous as anything I had experienced in my army training. Ordinarily, each cyclist would complete about ten miles or more on the flat, but the extraordinary winds meant that we could manage no more than three or four at a push. Back in the van after a stint, I stuffed myself with energy bars and high-calorie microwave meals, collapsed on to the fold-down bed for an hour or so and, dreading it, headed back into the wind howling across the prairie.

The route takes the cyclists through roughly 300 communities and occasionally, during the daylight hours, the traffic backed up behind. Except for the odd dickhead in a pick-up and a feed cap who'd honk his horn and tell us to go fuck ourselves, the Americans were incredibly friendly and encouraging all along the route. I was very touched when, at a changeover one morning, having just finished my leg, a woman crossed the street, congratulated us on our efforts and handed us a bag of McMuffins!

The first few days seemed to take forever, probably because we were slogging our way up the Rocky and Sierra mountains, but suddenly we were in Missouri and over the geographic halfway mark. By this stage we had caught up with the solo cyclists who set off three days ahead of the rest, cycling continuously for three days, eating on the hoof, stopping only to go to the toilet. Some of them were in such a state of exhaustion that they were wearing neck braces to keep their heads up. A little boil on my stomach that had been troubling me throughout the race seemed trifling by comparison. I had first noticed it in the final weeks of training and out in Orlando for the final settlement of the legal case. Self-diagnosing, I put it down to the zip on my Lycra cycling shirt, chafing against the skin. It wasn't a big deal, but it became irritating enough for me to start applying Trimovate antibacterial cream to it at increasingly frequent intervals.

The knowledge that the finishing line had become closer than the starting line acted like a shot of performance-enhancing drugs and two days later, the Appalachians behind us, we were bearing down on the finishing line. We arrived in the small hours, not expecting to see a soul but for an official with a clipboard, so it was very moving to be met by a crowd of about 100 clapping and whooping well-wishers as we crossed. We were still a few miles shy of Annapolis but it is there that the clock stops. We had crossed that vast continent in 7 days, 7 hours and 59 minutes at an average speed of 16.5mph, beating quite a number of the able-bodied teams and just behind a team of US vets who had six upright cyclists and two recumbents. From the finishing line, we were led into the beautiful port of Annapolis by a police escort and were greeted by another small but enthusiastic crowd. Far too tired to party right then, we headed for out cots and made up for it the next day.

After a day of rest and beers and hot meals, cooked in an oven and not in a microwave, our adventure came to an end with a visit to Washington, DC. The trip was organised by one of our sponsors, Anglo-American legal firm SNR Denton, and they had arranged for us to meet Senator John Kerry, a veteran of the Vietnam War. He was every bit as impressive as the reputation that preceded him and, perhaps because he too had been wounded, he seemed utterly sincere in his warmth towards us, making sure to stop and have a good chat with each of us.

The race organisers had given us a bag of goodies on completing the race, a medal and commemorative cycling shirt among the items. These are items that competitors cherish for the rest of their days, and during the training I had planned to send my shirt to Renee in Orlando as a gesture of thanks for all she had done for me, supreme proof of my recovery from my injuries. That opportunity, sadly, had gone and the shirt is still in its wrapper on a shelf in my cupboard at home.

32

Where my life had once been rooted in routine, just as I liked it, it had since taken on a slightly surreal and unpredictable quality, and I was starting to enjoy the richness, novelty and colour of the experiences that kept coming my way. The discipline and order of the army, the set timetables, the tight schedules, the immaculate kit and precision of work had been replaced by a pageantry of randomness I could never have imagined in my old life.

The dreamlike quality to my experiences at that time continued a couple of weeks after my return from the States when I found myself carrying the 2012 Olympic torch into Hemel Hempstead town centre. Unbeknown to me, my name had been put forward by several friends and I was bowled over to receive a letter telling me I would be carrying the torch on its final leg of the day, three weeks ahead of the opening ceremony in London. Dressed like a rapper in the baggy Olympic tracksuit and being unable to run, I walked as fast as my bilateral foot drop would allow through cheering crowds, among them my family and many friends I had known since childhood. Every step of the way I felt the honour of the opportunity that had been handed to me and, being a man not short on vanity, I lapped up the applause and the attention from the crowd and the cameras, with footage broadcast on news round-ups around the globe.

It was a dull, drizzly day but there were thousands of people lining the route, waving flags and cheering wildly, and I felt like the Pope on a foreign visit. Perhaps the policewoman escorting me was a radical Protestant because she seemed determined to stamp on the joy of the occasion by repeatedly telling me to hurry up and start running. I was powerwalking as fast as I could and at first I just smiled and ignored her, thinking the penny would drop and she would shut up. Evidently not. The fourth time she snapped at me, I rounded on her.

'This is me. This is all I can do. I have been chosen to carry this because of the wounds I have suffered. I can't bloody run! Geddit?'

It was the last I heard out of her but by then we were close to the finish and there was a fresh twist to the proceedings. A guy, no stranger to the tankard or so it appeared, erupted from the crowd and lurched towards me. I wasn't alarmed. One look at him and I knew I could have him. The thought crossed my mind that I might even take him down with a very un-Olympic swipe of the torch across his head. But he was grinning, a harmless happy pisshead, and as he reached me, he put a cigarette to his mouth, pointed at the flaming torch and asked me if didn't mind giving him a light. I saw the funny side of it, but he certainly wasn't laughing when a burly copper took him down with a rugby tackle.

It was a great day and I'll savour the memory of it forever, but I couldn't hang around for the festivities at the end of it. I had to be up at dawn the following morning to perform my first day's work since taking leave a few weeks before my accident in 2007. I was heading to Kenya, leading an expedition for 22 youngsters from a local secondary school. It was to be the first of eight expeditions I would take to exotic and challenging locations: Vietnam and Laos, Ecuador and Galápagos, Ethiopia, Borneo, India and two to the jungles of Central America. Each one was an adventure and a great responsibility, and I committed to them partly to earn a tiny bit of money, but mainly for the opportunity of putting something back, doing something to help others. I'd had quite enough of receiving kindness; the deficit column on the ledger of my conscience was showing I was deep in the red. These expeditions, using the skills I had learned in the army, were a small way of returning some of the goodness my world had shown to me.

In Kenya, we trekked through the Rift Valley, climbing to 4,000 metres, and to my great relief, there were no dramas. The only cause for anxiety was me, and the boil on my stomach that had troubled my biking across the States. It was annoying that it hadn't healed as quickly I thought once I got off the bike. If I'd known what I was to know in a few months' time, I would not have risked leading that expedition. Living in the wild, there was no guaranteed clean water to wash out the wound so I did the best I could with antiseptic creams, gauze and dressing. My field treatment had little effect, however, and by the time we landed back at Heathrow the protrusive lump of pus had doubled in size. The faint ring of alarm bells sounded deep in my mind. I had been so active in the last 15 months I had convinced myself that my recovery was all but complete. I didn't want to believe that anything could be seriously wrong with me. Again. Now that I had my life back, I just wanted to forge on with it.

33

It was a disgusting sight, this barely painful, weeping sore, a golf-ball-sized hole about two inches above where my belly button used to be. Gradually it took on the form of a living creature. I could feel it pulsing, like it had its own heartbeat, weeping, chafing, itching. A trained medic, I knew how to lance a boil and, fed the hell up with it one morning, I sterilised a needle over the gas hob and lanced the bastard. The fluid ran out, I covered it with Trimovate cream and applied a fresh dressing. Exhale. Job done.

But this boil wasn't giving up. Back it came with a vengeance, more furious than ever, and, through the pus, I could see the mesh holding back a ball of infection the size of a fist. I continued to treat it myself, but it just kept throbbing, like the vile creature inside John Hurt's stomach in *Alien*. I didn't want to spend one more day of my life in the company of a doctor or nurse – my problem, not theirs – but finally, grudgingly, I dragged myself up to the local surgery. Over the next few weeks, nurses cleaned and dressed it, but the little monster just stuck its head out further and further, the antibacterial and antifungal creams appearing to nourish not starve it of life.

On my umpteenth visit to the surgery, the stubborn bastard of a lump mocking my every stride into town, I lost my temper. Anger is what you get when anxiety and frustration boil over and mine burst out on the innocent girl tending to the suppurating ball of flesh throbbing out of my guts. It wasn't her fault the wound wasn't healing, that the system wasn't working. I demanded to see the GP and to his credit and my relief, he wrote out a letter there and then and told me to get myself down to A&E at Stoke Mandeville. To my surprise, I was ushered through to triage and seen within five minutes. To my dismay, the surgeon doing the seeing was Marwan Farouk, the one who had inserted the mesh in my second laparotomy two years earlier. He prodded and probed, turning his head this way and that. I could see that he was not happy about the spectacle before him, the rotten fruit of his labour, his manual labour. He told me I needed another laparotomy to re-mesh it. I said 'Fine' to his face and 'Fuck that for a game of soldiers' to myself as I stomped from the building.

I was stewing all the way home, at a complete loss as to who to turn to next. I was stuck in the system and the system said Marwan Farouk was going to carry out another life-or-death operation on me. You really don't want to undergo a single laparotomy if you can help it, let alone three. Farouk's first attempt obviously hadn't gone too well, so the prospect of letting him loose on my innards a second time was not a comforting one. Back home I started banging phones in the knowledge that, living off benefits and without private healthcare cover, my options were limited.

It was one of those happy coincidences in life that a few days later I found myself at a photoshoot at Bryan Adams's house in Chelsea. The Canadian rock singer and photographer was producing a book of powerful portraits of young British soldiers who had suffered life-changing injuries. *Wounded: The Legacy of War* aimed to raise awareness of the plight of severely injured personnel, and all the proceeds went to a raft of Armed Forces charities. It was fitting perhaps that it was there that I found the help I needed so desperately.

I spotted Linda Walton, the head of grants at Help for Heroes, and made a beeline for her. Another flesh-and-blood angel in my life, Linda was one of the few people I'd open up to about my problems and we had become good friends. Now, at the end of my wits and waiting in the wings for my turn before the camera, I unloaded on her, spilling my fears about going back to the same surgeon to have a repeat of the same meshing procedure that had led to me needing yet another massive operation. I lifted my shirt, she took a step back and covered her mouth – a dance routine I had seen many times during my recovery.

'Leave it to me,' she said. 'I know just the people to help resolve this.'

Thank you Bryan Adams, thank you Linda Walton. The next day, Linda called me at home with contact details for two surgeons, Rod Dunn and Alex Crick, who ran a war injuries clinic at Salisbury District Hospital. Linda had spoken to them and they were expecting my call. They were always incredibly busy, she said, but they were first-rate, compassionate surgeons and they were happy to take a look at me and see what they could do. I called and got Rod, and poured months of anxiety down the line. When I shut up, he said, 'When can you get down?'

'Tomorrow?'

It's a two-and-a-half-hour drive to Salisbury from Leighton Buzzard and I set off early. Within five minutes of checking in, I was being inspected by Rod, instantly reassured, before he had said anything of clinical note, just by his manner and outlook. He was cheerful and frank and, being an ex-Royal Marine, to him an obstacle was just a task to overcome before you cracked on to the next one. He went away and came back with Alex Crick. She was in the middle of an operation or heading into one, fully scrubbed up, and I could see only her eyes between face mask and surgical cap. I was lying on a gurney and, as she peered at the infection from all angles, I gabbled on about how it had been getting steadily worse for about six months.

'You need a CT scan so we can see exactly what's going on in there. What you see here is just the tip of the iceberg.'

'Christ, really? I've had enough radiation to last me a lifetime.'

'You need a CT scan.'

'Fine. So am I looking at having it meshed again?'

'No, I'd reconstruct you naturally, using sutures.'

I admitted I was confused about the best route: meshing or stitching. To my ignorant mind, meshing sounded like a more robust form of protection, like the stuff you use to cover battle tanks from enemy eyes or scaffolding from storm damage. Stitching is what your granny does in front of *Antiques Roadshow*.

'We can fit you in. We can help you try and sort this out. There are no cast iron guarantees in surgery, but I'd hope once and for all.'

I was really confused now. I took to Alex Crick as instantly as I had to Rod Dunn. She had an air of calm authority and goodness about her. But Farouk had been insistent that remeshing was the only option. Rod told me to go away and think about it for 24 hours – with the parting comment that Alex Crick was one of the best in the business and that they could oversee my recovery in the comforting surroundings of Tedworth House down the road.

I went home and started surfing the web. Dr Google, I had learned, is not the most reliable diagnostician. He knows everything and nothing. He loves to play with your head. He loves to show you how clever he is and how dumb you are. You can tell him what you really want, or really don't want, and he'll keep obliging you with whatever you want or do not want to hear. When I asked him what was better in a laparotomy, mesh or suture, he just said it cuts both ways, depends how you want to look at it, Jamie. Dr Fucking Google is the devil that speaketh with forked tongue, a cruel tyrant with a lot of smooth talk on him, and he's full of shit. He's got all the knowledge but none of the wisdom. The slippery, vindictive old bastard couldn't make his mind up about the better of the two procedures any more than I could. I snapped shut my laptop, slept on it and woke with a clear mind. I called Salisbury and spoke to Alex Crick.

It was a no brainer. Dunn and Crick filled me with confidence, Farouk filled me with dread. The mesh had palpably failed so why not give sutures a crack? The next week I was down in Salisbury being fed into the CT-scan pizza oven. My hopes higher than its famous spire, I left the cathedral city with a pocketful of powerful antibiotics to ward off the sepsis, and a promise to get me into theatre as soon as there was a space in Alex's rammed schedule – and a promise from me that, yes, in the meantime I'd contact her or Rod immediately, were the problem to get any worse. The idea was that the super-strong antibios would keep the spread of infection at bay until the op. Crick and Dunn – two names of a double act as comforting as Morecambe and Wise and Marks and Spencer – nonetheless left me in no doubt about the gravity of my condition. When I asked them if they really had to go through with it, hoping that there might be a non-invasive option, I was told: 'You need this operation or it's going to be the death of you.'

I had watched a laparotomy as a trainee patrol medic when, masquerading as a junior doctor, I was posted to one of the largest hospitals in southern England for a month. A woman had been stabbed 27 times by her boyfriend and I sat in on the team of surgeons battling to save her. Fascinated and appalled, I watched them cut her straight and deep down the middle, through the thick wall of muscle and fat, opening her up and peeling her back as wide as she'd go so they had all the space they needed to get to work on her, rummaging around in her vital organs like searching in a bag of shopping, the blood and blades glistening under the bright lights. I was in awe of these surgeons, so focused and determined in their work, and when they were done – incredibly she lived – they stitched her up with heavy sutures, her abdominal wall now like a tight Victorian corset. The operation went on for hours and hours, and I was transfixed throughout, all the time feeling so relieved that it was not me lying there, peeled back like a tin of sardines, with a gut full of latex gloves and tools. Now, barely six years later, I was about to undergo that same operation for a third time.

I was very nervous this time. Being in a coma, I knew nothing about my first laparotomy and, for the second, I was so desperate to get rid of the immense ball of hernia hanging off me that I would have had it done under local anaesthetic had that been the only option. But now, some serious happiness back in my life, so close to restoration, to my body being almost fully operational again, I was as anxious as I had ever been. Not depressed, just shitting myself. I had come so far but Fate had thrown one last massive obstacle in my path. It was a cruel, sick joke. Over the years of my recovery I had researched in depth every single condition with I had been afflicted and every procedure I had undergone (this was to be my sixty-first operation under general anaesthetic). I knew too well that the laparotomy was a major operation, highly distressing for the body. There's a limit to the surgical attrition it can endure, and a third excavation of my innards was sure to be the most gut-wrenching of the three. The ugly protrusion pushing itself out into the open was the outward proof that all was far from well on the inside. Alex Crick was going to have her hands in there for many hours.

I checked into Salisbury District on New Year's Day 2013, and it was fortunate that I was going to be catching up on my sleep over the coming days because it was an uneasy night, twisting and flopping from side to side. I was awake when the nurses came to me at dawn – and ravenous, but being nil-by-mouth, it would be some time before I'd get a solid meal inside me. I was wheeled down to theatre, and as the anaesthetist readied me for oblivion, I found myself saying a prayer in my head, something that I had not done since I was a child.

When it was all over, my eyes didn't spring open. For days, I lay in a haze, drifting in and out consciousness, aware only of excruciating pain and the ethereal movement of bodies around my bed. I had been told in the pre-op briefing that for two or three days the site would be left open, the abdominal wall and skin unstitched. Sponges soaked with strong antibiotics were to be pressed into the abdominal cavity and a vacu-pump attached to remove any incipient infection. On the fourth day, I was taken back to theatre and Alex Crick stitched me up with a single heavy tensile suture, for my very own corset.

I was kept in Salisbury for eight days and, just as Crick and Dunn had warned, the pain was appalling, the worst I had experienced since the flames in the cockpit. It was so great that I yelled and cried for many hours. I was also experiencing postoperative hypothermia, a common complication after major surgery. The combination of anaesthetic drugs and the exposure of my skin to the air for such a long period had resulted in a sharp drop of my core body temperature. I was wrapped in an electric heat blanket, but I still shuddered like I was having a fit. Thank God for painkillers. Most of the time I was completely out of it, especially for the first few days. Slowly, the pain subsided from unbearable to extreme, the analgesics were reduced a little, I stopped shaking with cold and I was awake for long enough periods to hold a groggy conversation.

Towards the end of the week, I was well enough for Alex Crick to talk me through what she done. She explained that the polymer mesh from the second 'lap' had become embedded, triggering inflammation and infection. Her task was straightforward, she said, but, I inferred, extremely painstaking. She had to pick out all the mesh, bit by tiny bit, and every last part of it, to be sure there would be no reinfection. The original mesh was about the size of a sheet of A4 paper so it would have been a back-breaking effort to pluck out the miniscule pieces enmeshed and stuck in the tissue and muscle. It took her half a day, bent forward under the bright lights picking away at the mess, a bowel surgeon on standby among the surgical team just in case. I am not embarrassed to admit that, after she left the ward, I wept with relief and gratitude for what she had done.

It takes months to recover from major invasive surgery like that and I spent the first three weeks of mine at Tedworth House, the superb recovery centre run by Help for Heroes. Situated 15 miles north of Salisbury, the seventeenth-century stately home, used as a club by US servicemen in the Second World War, Tedworth is about as fine a place imaginable for the severely wounded to recover. I was given my own room but as soon I was mobile enough to hobble I spent as much time as possible in the communal areas, watching TV and reading or, when I was feeling exhausted, which was often, dozing in an armchair gazing out over the stunning grounds.

I was eating normally by the time I left hospital and the food at Tedworth is the standard of a smart hotel. But it's the staff who make the experience such a heartening and uplifting experience, the pastoral care as good as you'll get anywhere. It was while I was there that I resolved to commit the next few years of my life to furthering the cause of that charity. I had been on the receiving end of so much kindness and goodwill for over five years, that I realised wasn't going to feel comfortable in my soul until I had given an equal amount of time back to those, like me, who really needed a helping hand.

It was a very cold period, that early January 2013, and one morning we woke to the magical sight of snow covering the lawns and sitting on the branches of the majestic old trees. I spent most of the time I was awake chatting to the other convalescents, many of them fighting their way back from hideous wounds sustained on the battlefield in Afghanistan. After all that training, at the very last moment, my opportunity to do my bit for Queen and Country had been snatched away – and that will always fester in me.

The thought crossed my mind many times, sitting there among new friends, many without legs and arms, that maybe I would have ended up in Tedworth House anyhow. I didn't envy them, but it hurt that they had sustained their wounds with honour and I regretted that mine had come as a result of some idiot who had failed to put enough oil in the engine or tighten a wing nut securely enough. I could take only a little pride from the knowledge that it was probably my army training that had saved my life – all those drills, that striving for perfection, the coolness under intense pressure that they drum into you.

Looking out over that winter landscape, I could feel proud that five years earlier, sitting in raging flames for just under a minute, I had brought in the aircraft, just as the emergency protocol had instructed. I turned off every switch, took the decision to veer away from the skull-cracking, back-breaking asphalt, climb on to the wing, my body on fire, waited in the blasting flames fanned by the propeller and, just at the right moment, neither a second too early nor too late, jump to earth and give myself the smallest chance of living.

I took a slurp from my mug of tea and went back to *Diver* magazine. It's not much to feel proud about, but you take what you can in this life.

Afterword

The recovery from my laparotomy was going to take three months and, back home from Tedworth House, there was little I could do each day but sit in an armchair, read books and, from time to time, head outside to build up my mobility. Doubled up, I had to do this very gingerly for the first few weeks, walking up and down Mum's street, just as I had done after Farouk's effort, then branching a little further afield into Leighton Buzzard. When I graduated to the next level and set out into the surrounding hills, I knew that Alex Crick's epic work in the Salisbury operating theatre had fixed me for life.

After 120 operations and procedures, constant illness and pain, I had developed an acutely sensitive intuition into the state of my body. Every throb, twitch, spasm, bolt, stab and itch told its own little story. I could read my body like a book. Long before I was fully healed, I just knew I was going to be okay, that this time I was sorted for good, that I no longer needed to fret about my health any more than the person next to me on the bus. Six years after feeling the first flames of the engine fire licking around my ankles, I had been given my life back.

Alex Crick considers the operation she performed on me as just something she did that day, an appointment in her busy schedule that week. She has performed hundreds of major operations. I have seen her a couple of times since and she shrugs about it. It's just a day's work for her. This is partly her modesty, partly the magic of surgery that is slightly lost on the people who do it for a living, but never on the patients whose lives have been restored by their skills and tenacity. For me, the third laparotomy was a key milestone in my life, triggering a miraculous and permanent transformation, as much in my outlook as in my physical capabilities. When Alex Crick ran the final suture through the skin of my abdomen, she gave me closure in every sense.

I have had a number of procedures on my skin since, mainly to my face, including pioneering laser and stem cell work performed at the Harley Street Skin Clinic. I am still having it today and it is carried out by Aamer Khan, a brilliant cosmetic surgeon and a good guy who does a lot of charity work. For most people, each one of these procedures would be a massive ordeal. My face is always red and raw, and it hurts like hell for a few days, like extreme sunburn with a lemon squeezed over it. I'm not getting all SAS-macho on you when I say that, for me, it's no big deal. Pain and suffering are relative and, inevitably after all my grim experiences, my agony threshold had become pretty high.

Besides, pain is easier to withstand if you know for sure that good will flow from it. A great deal of good has flowed from my trips every three months to see Dr Khan. After each procedure, once it has settled down, I look in the mirror and see that my face has improved. People no longer turn away in horror or embarrassment these days. Their eyes may linger that little bit longer, but that's just curiosity, not sympathy or disgust. They want to know the story. In their face, each time I see the same question: *Poor guy, I wonder what happened to him?* I'm fine with that. I like that connection, the passing engagement with a fellow human being, me going my way, them going theirs trying to figure out what the hell had happened, maybe wondering how I was feeling about it, what my life was like as a result.

I can tell how far I have come by the reaction of women. Women are better at looking beyond the superficial appearance to the inner being. If a woman had a face like mine, no guy would look at her. Men are crap like that. For most guys, beauty is just about looks and figures. Girls are more interested in character so once in a while, when I get a smile from a woman on the street or on the train, I am moved and uplifted by the gesture. They can see I'm doing okay, that I'm getting on with it, that I'm happy with myself again.

I am not going to bore you with every last event that has happened since Alex Crick gave me my life back, but suffice to say I have done a great deal! I have been skydiving, I have qualified as a hot-air balloon pilot, I have competed in the Invictus Games, I have bought a small apartment in London. This has given me a sense of independence as I ready myself to start a new career, whatever that might prove to be. I have overcome my deepest fears and taken to the air in a light aircraft. But for the most part, I have cycled, walked, talked and run my smelly socks off, all for charity.

The most satisfying effort has been biking from John o'Groats to Windsor in memory of Fusilier Lee Rigby, slaughtered by savages on a London street on a spring day in 2013. I had met Lee's father, Phil McClure, at a Help for Heroes talk I gave to employees of haulage firm Eddie Stobart where he works as one of their long-distance drivers. Phil is a lovely guy and I felt an instant and deep connection with him, the grief of his son's hideous death etched into his face like it had been sculpted. When I went away, I came up with a plan: to cycle in Lee's memory and raise money for Help the Heroes, with Phil acting as our support driver.

I cycled with my friend Jonathan Trafford and it was a stunning ride, with Phil doing an outstanding job as our support man. The Scottish Highlands are a tough challenge to navigate on a bike and Traf and I would have been completely lost without him. It was emotional too, thinking of Lee and Phil all along the route, a strange experience for me, feeling the sympathy, not receiving it. The Scots were great, their kindness and generosity lifting our morale all the way. Our van was decorated with Help for Heroes banners and every time we stopped at a café for a coffee or a sandwich, without any invitation the locals came over and dropped money into the collection buckets. On two occasions, we found that our bill had been settled by strangers. It's experiences like those that make you get the point of it all, make you forget the slog it can be.

As in my earlier life, when I was fully able-bodied, it has all been about reaching goals that I felt were close to or just beyond my reach. The body may be broken, but a strong spirit doesn't limp or quail. Mine is in good fettle and, if anything, I have pushed myself harder than ever. The peaks to which I have ascended may have been lower, but the effort just as great, perhaps greater.

Walking had been the principal vehicle of my rehabilitation as an outpatient and, surprise, surprise, I had become obsessed by it, pushing myself to take on ever longer distances. I began to hunt out the biggest walking events out there, but at the back of my mind I knew there was only one challenge for me – the hardest one I could find! The International Four Days Marches in Nijmegen, in the Netherlands, is one of the toughest out there and, after proving I could run a marathon, my old mate and dive buddy Gary 'Gaz' Jones began bending my ear about us doing it together. With 200km to cover in four days, it is not an event for the leaden-footed or the faint-hearted and you need to go into training to stand a chance.

To test my capabilities, we entered the inappropriately named 'Dorset Doddle', a 50-kilometre one-day event, walking from Weymouth to Swanage over gruelling terrain, up and down a precipitously steep coastal path. I found it utterly shattering and it was especially hard because I still had an abdomen full of infection. (It was a couple of months before the third laparotomy that got rid of it.) Despite Gaz's chirpy banter keeping me upright, I literally staggered over the finishing line at five in the morning, four hours after the cut-off point to get the official badge. A failure on paper, but a massive triumph all the same.

I don't like failing to meet a challenge and Nijmegen continued to taunt me. In 2017, five years after the 'Dorset Doddle', the pull was too great and I found myself on a flight to the Netherlands, desperate to take part in this famous walk. You walk 50k for four straight days over asphalt roads, tracks and paths and, like the great marathons, it is a fabulous experience and atmosphere, half of Holland either participating or lining the route and cheering wildly. It is not a competition, so the vibe is communal, like a giant party on the move. I was thrilled to complete the first day but, drained to the marrow and blistering, I pulled off my shoes and collapsed on to the bed. When the alarm went off at 4am the next morning, I could barely make it to the bathroom I was so stiff. I watched days two and three on my hotel television with my feet in a bowl of hot water and Epsom salts, but on the fourth, still aching, I dragged my weary arse and tender feet to the start line and, 14 hours later, I fell punch-drunk over the finishing line. The smiling crowds were roaring with glee, the flags waving, but unlike Dorset, Nijmegen felt like a failure. I wasn't done trying yet. I had to return.

Two years later, I was back, lost amidst the joyful throng, bigged up all the way round by my fellow participants. That summer of 2019 was one of the hottest on record and we walked every day in a heatwave, guzzling water and energy drinks. It wasn't about the medal. It never is. It was about being able to live with myself. That may sound daft to many, but I have demons to slay, always have done and, able-bodied or disabled, I have to keep putting them to the sword. At Nijmegen, I slayed the full dragon.

For me, life without overcoming challenges is not worth living, always has been, always will be.

• • •

I have thrown myself back into my life, trying to make up for the lost years of my prime, helped and encouraged by some extraordinarily good people. That's the greatest legacy of a severe life-changing accident like mine – you discover there is an awful lot of kindness, goodwill and sacrifice out there. I may never have known that otherwise, or at least never fully understood quite how much decency and nobility is hidden away in the souls of fellow travellers on life's stony path. It's been very heartening and enlightening. I wouldn't go so far as to say that gaining this new awareness makes being torched to the bone worth it, but it's certainly been a surprising bonus of my experience. I have come to understand myself better as a result of this awakening. I realise now that in my drive to make myself a better person, to make something of my life after a shaky start, I had become self-obsessed to the point of selfishness. I allowed very little to stand in my way in my push to the top. Today, I understand that we only reach these peaks with the love and support of family and friends, the encouragement of colleagues and, in my case, the incredible work of medics and, just occasionally, the miraculous, Samaritan intervention of total strangers.

It is for this reason, not for guilt, not for settling debts of kindness, not for want of anything better to do, that I have given so much of my life since my recovery in working as an ambassador for the charity Help for Heroes. Yes, they gave me incredible help when I needed it and, yes, they gave me experiences I shall never forget and would never have enjoyed otherwise. But their greatest gift to me has been the opportunity to do unto others as others have done unto me. By giving my time to their cause, I have not been fulfilling a moral obligation, not executing my duties in an unwritten contract – I have been doing what comes naturally to someone who has been the recipient of so much kindness himself. I have *wanted* to help others. I have *needed* to do it.

I have lost count of all the talks I have given to august institutions, businesses, societies and schools. I have told my story and the lessons I have learned from it over and over, bored daft by the sound of my own voice, but in doing so I hope I have managed to communicate the possibility in all of us of growing as a character from the scorching furnace of a dreadful experience. Above all, I hope I have communicated the importance of showing kindness – an importance impossible to measure – to those who suffer. That kindness need not be expressed only in grand gestures like serious charity work, or major events like life-saving surgery, or a mother at her son's bedside for months on end. It can, as I discovered, be expressed in the little gestures. One person's happiness can be built up by the accumulation of a thousand small offerings of goodwill – Renee talking to me in my coma, Matt Hawkes giving up his suppers to come and sit with me, Pete Mash beasting me up a mountain, Des Stockdale getting me a place on the London Marathon, the smiling newsagent pretending he sees nothing wrong with my disfigured face ... I could list a thousand and more such acts that, gesture by gesture, have helped restore my love of life, my faith in my fellow man.

Building a new life from the ground up – from where I lay burning in the long grass, seconds from death – has been a long and painstaking ordeal, the gradient of my recovery graph very shallow, nudging along the horizontal axis, the occasional upward spike among many dips back towards the bottom. The graph peaks sharply at the time of Pastor Billy's extraordinary intervention and during the month I spent with Pete Mash in Colorado and then, during that manic 18 months of marathons, cycling and winter sports, it takes on the impression of a mountain range, a very graphic representation indeed of my lust for life, my urgency to be me again. But the angle of the line, marking my overall state of well-being, still ran fairly low and flat. It is only after the surgery in Salisbury that the line turns markedly upwards and begins to climb steeply.

I was an elite soldier, now I have a Disabled blue badge. That hurts a little still, mainly because, after all the punishing effort to get to the top of my profession, I never got to test myself where it really matters: in a combat zone. But that's a minor moan, barely worth the effort of making it. I'm as proud of my recovery as I am of anything I have ever achieved. I needed way more resilience to get through those five hard years than anything I have ever undertaken – and once again I can do most of the things that I used to take for granted, just not to the same levels. You'd probably beat me in a 100-yard dash or a marathon, but hey, I'd likely hammer you in a bike ride up in the hills!

As my capabilities improved, there remained one gaping hole in my life – scuba diving. I tried blocking it out, deleting the daydreams as they appeared in my head, but it got sneaky on me and started appearing in my dreams at night: me slipping beneath the surface of the water into that strange and magical world, another dimension altogether, as far removed from daily life on earth as floating through the stratosphere in a space capsule. After all that I have regained in my life, bemoaning the loss of scuba diving may sound like a churlish gripe, the wail of a spoilt child who wants everything. But diving was my great passion. For some, it might be hillwalking or playing the piano, going to the theatre or riding their Harley, collecting vintage stamps or growing orchids, dinghy sailing or birdwatching. For me, it has always been scuba diving that has brought the greatest joy in life. It was my refuge, my retreat, my chance to feel wonder.

I missed it terribly. I was convinced I would never again have that sensation of ducking beneath the waves and sinking happily into the deep, leaving all my troubles up above, the glow of it staying with me for hours and days afterwards.

So, my heart sunk when the phone rang and it was Theresa Simpson, my friend and former PADI course director who I had worked for at Emperor Divers in Egypt all those years ago. Hearing about my accident through the dive community she was keen to help me out in any way she could, saying I need only pick up the phone and she'd arrange a trip for me, all paid for by Emperor. It was a lovely gesture, but I explained ruefully that, my body being compromised now, I probably lacked the strength and mobility to dive safely and that I was worried about the effect on my still fragile skin. It could even be dangerous, I said, not just for me but my dive buddy if, say, we were to find ourselves in a strong current or there was a malfunction with the kit. She pointed out that the saltwater might actually be good for my skin and, as reassurance, they would make sure I went down with a highly experienced diver. The memories were seeping back as we spoke, the temptation mounting and it wasn't too long before I heard myself saying, 'What the hell? You only go round once.' As she said, once in the water, I'd know pretty quickly whether I was up to it and, if I wasn't, there was nothing to stop me getting straight back out. No one was going to wrestle me to the seabed. So a few weeks later I found myself on a flight to Hurghada, the anxieties swarming in my guts the closer we got to Egypt.

Even in the baking heat of the Red Sea, the water can be freezing cold at low depths and your dive suit should always be as tight as a drum on the body to prevent it getting in and forcing down your core body temperature to dangerous levels. It's hard enough wriggling and yanking yourself into a wetsuit at the best of times, the neoprene scrubbing over the skin. When the liveaboard boat reached the dive site and the big moment had arrived I was every bit as nervous as I had been making my first parachute jump. I don't usually lack for courage – and I was a Master Instructor for God's sake – but my confidence was shot. I felt like a little kid on my first day at school – and the good thing about a wetsuit is that you can piss your pants and no one will know.

My old dive buddy, Gaz Jones, picked up on my anxiety and came over to help me into the suit and we managed eventually to get it on without ripping open my skin or so much as nicking it. I strapped on my weights belt and buoyancy jacket (BCD), heaved the 33-pound scuba tank on to my back, the straps digging hard into my collarbone. I ran through my checks, my heart revving in overdrive, and I took some deep, slow breaths through my nose, punching them out, trying to hide my fears from the others, throwing some plastic smiles, the boat rocking wildly in the swell. They were polite enough to pretend they hadn't noticed, but I could tell they all knew I was virtually soiling myself.

Sliding our masks on to our heads and stepping into our fins, we slapped our way to the open board at the stern of the boat. Mohammed, the dive leader, and the other two stepped straight into the water one after the other, easy as falling off a log, and quickly resurfaced, their faces bobbing in the swell like seals. I stood on the board, legs apart, arms out at the side desperately trying to keep my balance, a great lump of nerves in my throat. I felt exactly as I had before taking the plunge for my first ever dive about 20 years earlier.

'Come on in, Jamie, the water's fine!'

I put my hand over my mask, took a giant stride and, breaking the water, sank like a boulder. Electrified by panic and exhilaration, it was a couple of seconds before I found the inflator button and thumbed it to get some more air into my BCD. The jacket tightened sharply around my chest and I rocketed to the surface, spewing water from the back of my mouth and gulping the scorching hot air. I rose and fell in the strong swell, clearing the salty water from my nostrils and adjusting my mask, trying not to bite so damned hard on the rubber mouthpiece of my regulator.

Mohammed made the okay sign – it was a question not a statement and I returned the gesture, answering in the affirmative but feeling anything but okay. Their heads disappeared, and I was left treading the water, my stomach muscles straining with the effort of keeping clear of the boat. I took a huge breath, dumped the air in my BCD and slid beneath the waves, the noises above instantly muffled, my limbs floating in slow motion like a space-man, entirely out of kilter with the speed of my bolting heart. I slid towards the darkness, the warped noise from the boat now a faint hum. We paused at five metres, finning on the spot, facing each other in a circle.

Mohammed pointed in the direction of a hazy reef, a dark blur in the distance, and we all made the okay gesture and pushed away alongside him. The cold increased as we made our way down, my breathing began to slow, my heart rate to settle and I started to look around. When you're nervous underwater, fretting about your equipment or your buddy, you don't take in the surroundings so well. I was fretting less about my kit and more about my physical capabilities, the reaction of my body to the ever-heavier atmospheric pressure, the salt on my skin. Was I making a terrible mistake, putting mine and other lives at risk here? But with every metre we descended, with every flick of the fin, the anxiety gave way to relief and the relief to joy, a joy soon unravelling faster than the rope of a heavy anchor.

Hundreds of multicoloured fish darted among the waving vegetation of the reef, the fractured light of the sun, so glaring on the surface, now suffusing the scene with a warm mellowness. A ray wriggled on the pure white sand of the sea floor, stirring up little plumes of the finest particles. We stopped above the reef and formed another circle. Mohammed pointed to me and, making the okay gesture again and tilting his head, he was asking me how I was getting on. I stabbed back my own okay, clenched my fists like I was celebrating a goal, and broke into a grin so wide my mouthpiece popped out. He returned the smile and throwing out an open hand, offered me to take the lead.

Yeah, I can do that! I pointed downwards towards the rough shape of another mountainous reef off the starboard of the boat. I swished my fins and suddenly I was out in front, sliding through a great shaft of opaque sun, like the light through a cathedral window, back in my element, chasing that happiness.

Acknowledgements

I wish to acknowledge the mountain of support I received from my ghostwriter, Niall Edworthy, in his help crafting this book – a uniquely challenging and significant process between us both, which took over two years of dedicated research to conclude.

I would like to thank my editor, Lorna Russell at Ebury Press, Penguin Random House Group, for all her valuable input and professional advice towards publication.

I also wish to acknowledge and thank Bethany Wright at Ebury Press, who diligently helped to compile and choreograph the detailed image section.

A special mention also goes to my Senior Literary Agent, Annabel Merullo at Peters, Fraser and Dunlop, for her genuine understanding of my journey, and for believing in the power and reach of my story.

Photo credits

Plate section images:

p1, bottom left: Adam Smith-Connor

p2, top left: Orlando Regional Health Centre, Florida, USA

p3, top: Dr Paul M. Smith, Cardiff Metropolitan University

p4, top: Help for Heroes veterans' charity www.helpforheroes.org.uk

p4, bottom: Dr Sandy Saunders, for and on behalf of all the Guinea Pig Club members

p5, bottom: Flight examiner Brian George Jones OBE

p6, middle: Sue Foulds

p6, bottom: Blesma veterans' charity www.blesma.org

p7, top: Jonathon Daniel Pryce www.garconjon.com

p7, bottom: Niall Edworthy

p8, top: Lieutenant Colonel Andy Reid

p8, bottom: Joanne Mildenhall

With thanks to Blesma, The Limbless Veterans for permission to use their photograph on the front cover.

Blesma, The Limbless Veterans was formed in the years following the First World War and became a national charity in 1932. Blesma is dedicated to assisting serving and ex-Service men and women who have experienced loss of limb, use of limbs, hearing, sight or speech, either during or after service. We support these men and women and their families in their communities throughout the UK and overseas.